"The first thing that comes to my mind when reading this book is passion! A person who lives his life by the truest meaning of a martial artist. With so much detail throughout the book the author breaks down the science behind fighting and the techniques that are required to become a complete stand up confident martial artist-fighter.

This book will give a complete beginner with no martial arts knowledge or experience to a seasoned professional fighter the steps of scientific movement and correct form.

As a former 11x World Muay Thai Champion I would recommend this book to all martial artist and beginners to upgrade their skills and true understanding of technique form and why karate is a powerful way of life"

Nathan Carnage Corbett

11 time World Muay Thai Champion

HARD CONTACT KARATE
Karate secrets for full contact fighting

Copyright © 2020 by Paul Jackman

ISBN 978-1-7771106-0-4

All rights reserved. No part of this publication may be reproduced, distributed, or transmitted in any form or by any means, including photocopying, recording, or other electronic or mechanical methods, without the prior written permission of the publisher, except in the case of brief quotations embodied in critical reviews and certain other noncommercial uses permitted by copyright law.

The information in this book is meant to supplement, not replace, proper Karate training. Like any sport involving speed, equipment, balance and environmental factors, Karate poses some inherent risk. The authors and publisher advise readers to take full responsibility for their safety and know their limits. Before practicing the skills described in this book, be sure that your equipment is well maintained, and do not take risks beyond your level of experience, aptitude, training, and comfort level.

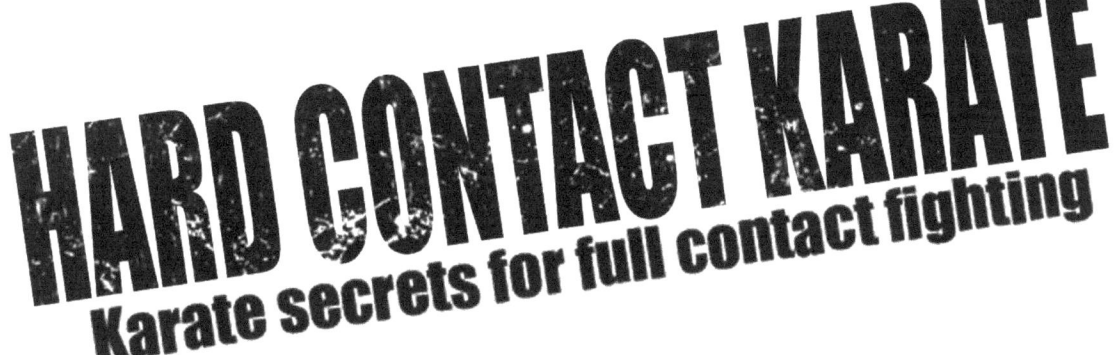

Paul Jackman 7th Dan

4 Time World Koshiki Contact Karatedo Champion

FOREWORD

KARATE PRINCIPLES AND TECHNIQUES FOR CONTACT FIGHTING

<u>Secrets for success in and out of the ring</u>

Karate originated as a Budo Art from Okinawa, meant to fight without weapons. Honouring this origin, Koshiki Contact Karate-do is a systematic fighting method using bare hands and feet! Like any other combative art, this practice also requires challenging work and sweat, along with other fundamental ingredients such as commitment, discipline, patience, perseverance, courage, indomitable spirit and most importantly, access to elevated level coaching! Therefore, it is not surprising that these traits apply to any high-end art or discipline. By necessity, they are in fact the universal ingredients required to develop competent real-life fighting skills!

In fact, all of the above-mentioned characteristics have been pursued fully by World Koshiki Contact Karatedo champion (lightweight division) Shihan Paul Jackman 7th Dan. Rising as a lad, from the rough and ready back blocks of Trinidad, migrating to Canada to search for a functional style and eventually landing almost accidently, in a Shorinjiryu Kenkokan Karatedo dojo, Paul Jackman through his relentless effort, determination, and conviction to one day be a world champion in karate, did just that; he became a world champion, not once but four times!

As a previous (retired) coach, official, international tournament promoter, and World Koshiki Contact Karatedo Executive Member, Shihan Paul had the pleasure of watching this karate warrior progress from fighting his way (literally) onto the Canadian International Koshiki team that competed at the world titles in Australia in 2000. Then, he went onto competing at various International Koshiki competitions around the globe, where over the next decade and a half Shihan Paul eventually fought his way to the top of his game. He consistently won in kata and kumite at these events. His speed, technical acumen, and fierce competitive spirit became legendary amongst the international Koshiki fighter's fraternity.

While Shihan Paul developed as a fighter and competitor, he also morphed into a top referee, coach, and dojo operator who earned his way onto the international executive committee for his chosen combative sport and discipline. Today, Shihan Paul is one of the international leaders of 'the next generation' very ably representing Canadian Koshiki Contact Karate, including becoming a successful promoter of his art. This experience and more, is captured in his book 'Karate Principles and Techniques For Contact Fighting'. I found his book to be a great read, informative, indeed instructional! All the aspects covered in this book are fundamental to becoming a successful 'stand up' fighter. This book also touches on other relevant elements to Shorinjiryu Kenkokan Karatedo, the Kudaka/Hisataka family style of Japan based Okinawan karate, and World Koshiki Contact Karatedo, headed by Masayuki Kudaka Hanshi 10th Dan and Masamitsu Kudaka Hanshi 8th Dan, both of whom are Shihan Paul's instructors.

This book serves as an excellent guide to effective punching, kicking, and striking and is written in straight talk! I highly recommend it for any karate athlete and practitioner!

Nigel McReaddie

8th Dan Shihan, Kenryukan Karate-jutsu

Brisbane, Queensland, Australia

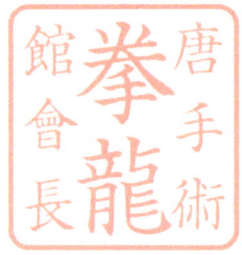

ABOUT THE AUTHOR

MY NAME IS Paul Jackman and since a young age, I have been obsessed with martial arts. My journey in martial arts started at the age of 9 on the island of Trinidad where I grew up. Being a small guy growing up in a tough place, I realized at a young age that I needed to be able to defend myself. I hated the feeling of being afraid of other people and not being in control of that fear. As a young boy, I was exposed to Japanese culture and martial arts via two of my childhood best friends who came from Japanese diplomatic families. It was from these early life experiences that my love for martial arts, especially Japanese Budo really took roots. At the same time, I have always been a very logical and scientific thinker. From an early age, I understood the difference between ideas that are good in theory and ideas that would work in practice. I had a strong understanding and awareness that ideas need to be tested in realistic conditions to determine their effectiveness. It is safe to say that throughout my martial arts career I have always been interested in those arts that are scientifically sound and have been tested in the real world.

In the mid 1990's, I moved to Canada and as a young man I was anxious to train hard and test myself in the most realistic ways. In the back of my mind, I always had the question "Would this work in a real-life situation?" As I began to advance my training in martial arts, my personal philosophy was that every technique and training method I learned had to stand up to this scrutiny. I explored many dojos and styles looking for a place to train and found that the training practices in most places seemed rigid, robotic, and not very practical. At the same time, most training places did not place much focus on actual fighting and those that did had turned sparing and fight training into a modified game of tag. As such, even with limited traditional training, I could see that what was being preached at these places would not be of much help in a real-life situation. In fact, in many cases, these techniques and moves could actually be detrimental if used in an uncontrolled non-theoretical environment.

After months of checking dojos and being disappointed with what I saw, I had almost given up on practicing a Traditional Japanese art in Canada. I began to think about starting boxing or kick boxing or even a contact fighting sport that seemed to be more popular in Canada. However, by luck or karma or maybe a combination of both, I happened to meet a man named Hubert O'Brien in a pub shooting pool who had a Karate emblem on his shirt. Due to our mutual interest in the martial arts, I began to engage in a conversation with him. Upon asking him a few questions, he told me that he taught at a small dojo just next door. I found this to be very ironic as I had been to this pub many times and hadn't even noticed the karate school just two doors down. He invited me to come and check it out sometime. He was not pushy and did not make an attempt for a big sales pitch but rather just gave me a friendly invitation to come and try it out. The styles he taught were known as Shorinjiryu Kenkokan and Koshiki Karatedo.

I accompanied him to the karate school and from the moment I stepped in, I knew I had found what I was looking for. The dojo was filled with hard armor like chest guards. I saw that people inside the dojo were smashing each other back and forth with thunderous punches and kicks. I was particularly impressed by their effortless moves as they delivered their punches and kicks while avoiding those coming at them. Soon after that, I registered to take classes at that location. My first class involved a detailed breakdown of the basic punching and kicking techniques, everything from foot positions to body mechanics in a very detailed and scientific manner that rang bells with everything I had learned about science, particularly physics in school.

As I mentioned above, I had found my martial arts home and soon learned that the style I was being taught came directly from Japan. In fact, I also discovered that the son of its founder Masayuki Kukan Hisataka was still alive and was actively teaching martial arts in Japan and internationally. At the time, he was actively involved in spreading the Koshiki karate fighting competition all over the world. World championship competitions were also held every couple of years to further promote this art on a global platform. I now felt even more inspired and determined to one day become his student and have an opportunity to directly train under him and perhaps one day even become a World champion in Koshiki Fighting.

In 2000, after many years of training with discipline and dedication, I qualified for the Canadian National Team to compete at my first World Koshiki Karate Championships held in Australia. I was also very excited to learn that I would have an opportunity to meet my role model at the championship, who later became my teacher and lifelong mentor.

This first experience changed my life not because I won a medal but because I skillfully responded to a good pounding at that tournament. I was also struck by the level of talent at the competition and was left in awe of the champions I saw that day. Moreover, my time at the championship gave me a taste of what it takes to be a champion and I became even more determined to reach that level.

Since that first world championship, I have won 4 world Koshiki karate championships in the light weight division (at 63.5 kg) and have achieved the rank of 6th Dan by Hanshi Masayuki Hisataka, 9th Dan himself. In 2007, I did a professional Mixed Martial Arts (MMA) exhibition match against one of Canada's top ranked bantam weights and demonstrated that traditional karate techniques can be used to a great effect in the MMA arena.

Hence, I believe very strongly that regardless of where one chooses to test themselves, whether in MMA, Kick Boxing, or any other contact fighting art, the secret lies in developing a systematic and overall understanding of all aspects related to fighting from technique to movement and timing to strategy. Furthermore, mental factors such as fear, determination, and fortitude also play an important role. In this book, I will present a detailed and systematic breakdown of all karate techniques and will share the concepts and strategies to be successful in a real testing ground.

PURPOSE OF THIS BOOK

REGARDLESS OF THE martial arts style, the ingredients required to develop competent real life fighting skills are somewhat universal. It is important that a martial artist builds their craft on a foundation of solid principals and an understanding of how these principals work and how they can be further developed. Body mechanics and movements must be understood as they relate to each technique. In this way, one can learn to use their whole body when executing any technique thereby, maximizing power and speed while achieving maximum effect with minimum effort. Through this unifying involvement of the whole body into a specific effort, one's actions and movements become more natural to their body and more efficient. Proper punching and kicking is not a natural thing for the human body so one must train for the use of proper techniques so as to make what is intuitively unnatural feel natural. This is precisely the meaning of the phrase: "Martial arts training can create unification with nature."

In addition to the many technical skills necessary to be successful in a real fighting situation, there are some equally important mental, emotional, and spiritual skills that must be developed in order to achieve success is any contact fighting arena. A fighter must be mentally prepared to deal with the high stress and chaotic atmosphere of fighting. A fighter must also be able to control the emotional responses to being hit so as to remain calm and be able to make strategic decisions. Mental and emotional responses tend to cause the body to tense up, making the fighter unable to react. For this reason, contact is extremely important in training and sparing. For this purpose, I highly recommend the use of bogu to facilitate very realistic contact training that helps sharpen one's techniques and also gets one used to being hit. This will allow a trainee to learn how to receive powerful strikes and at the same time control their emotional and mental responses that can be detrimental to success.

Another important factor is commonly known as "spiritual development", not in a religious sense, but in the sense of one's spirit or character. Their inner desire to push through adversity, to get up after being knocked down, and to succeed no matter how difficult or impossible the task. This kind of strength of spirit can only be achieved by constantly testing oneself in realistic combat, reevaluating one's techniques, and always looking for improvement. In this way, we say "spiritual development of mind and body" is crucial for a fighter's success.

With this book, it is my purpose and intent to give a complete account of the karate philosophy, technique, and strategy as they apply to the development of any contact martial artist. The following chapters, illustrations, and accompanying videos will give a full technical and scientific breakdown of the most common striking techniques, how to develop them, and how to put them all together to develop a solid strategy for success.

CONTENTS

Foreword ix
Karate Principles and Techniques for Contact Fighting ix
About the Author xi
Purpose of this book xv

Introduction 1
    Historical context: where does the practice of budo comes from? What is the difference with other forms of martial arts? 1
    Shorinjiryu kenkokan karatedo and koshiki karatedo. 2

Chapter 1: Developing The Mind, Body, and Spirit 5
    1.1 Why does one need to know how to fight? Why train in budo? 5
    1.2 An effective formula for learning 6
    1.3 Breathing, training, and fighting 7
    1.4 Learning the concept and not only the technique 9

Chapter 2: Stances, Postures, Movements, and Distancing 11
    2.2.1 Natural stance (shizentai dachi) 13
    2.2.2 Front stance (zenkutsu dachi) 14
    2.2.3 Back stance (kokutsu dachi) 15
    2.2.4 Cat stance (neko ashi dachi) 15
    2.2.5 Crane stance (tsuru ashi dachi) 16
    2.2.6 Open defensive stance (sotobiraki jigo hontai dachi) 17
    2.2.7 The fighting stance (fighting posture) 17
    2.3.1 Distancing 18
    2.3.2 Movement 19
    2.3.3 Types of steps 19
    2.3.4 Positioning movements 27
    2.3.5 Building footwork and movement 28

Chapter 3: Punching, Kicking, and Striking 29
    3.3.1 Straight punching techniques 33
    3.3.2 Shomen tsuki (the front punch - punching from a natural stance) 37
    3.3.3 Choku tsuki (straight punch, jab, or punching with the lead hand). 38
    3.3.4 Hineri tsuki (twist punch, reverse punch, cross or punching with the back hand). 40
    3.4.1 Straight kicks 43
    3.4.2 Roundhouse kicks 54
    3.4.3 Striking techniques 63
    Chapter summary 97

Chapter 4: Offensive Fighting..99
    4.1.1 Hand kuzushi (off-balancing by attacking the arms or guard) 100
    4.1.2 Kuzushi with the front hand...100
    4.1.3 Kuzushi from opposite stance to the opponent (eg. Left stance to right stance) 101
    4.1.4 Kuzushi with the back hand 103
    4.2.1 Inside leg checks..106
    4.2.2 Outside leg check...107
    4.4.1 Changing targets..110
    4.4.2 Changing weapons 110
    4.4.3 Changing direction of attack..110
    4.6.1 Leading with the hands 111
    4.6.2 Leading with the feet 113
    4.7.1 Leading with the hands 118
    4.7.2 Leading with the feet 120

Chapter 5: Defensive Fighting 127
    5.3.1 Neko ashi (cat step escape, front side escape) 128
    5.3.2 Hiraki ashi (open leg step, turning escape) 129
    5.3.3 Oi ashi (lunge escape, switching escape) 130
    5.3.4 Sankaku ashi (triangle step) 130
    5.3.5 Straight in escape 131
    5.5.1 Countering with a different weapon 132
    5.5.2 Countering with a different direction 133
    5.5.3 Countering at a different level 133
    5.6.1 Gonosen: countering after the attack (post attack) 133
    5.6.2 Tainosen: countering at the same time of the attack (simultaneous) 134
    5.6.3 Sennosen: countering just before the attack (pre-emptive) 134

Chapter 6: Strategies (putting it all together) 137
    6.7.1 Physical strength 140
    6.7.2 Cardiovascular fitness 141
    6.7.3 Flexibility 142

INTRODUCTION

HISTORICAL CONTEXT: WHERE DOES THE PRACTICE OF BUDO COMES FROM? WHAT IS THE DIFFERENCE WITH OTHER FORMS OF MARTIAL ARTS?

BACK IN THE mid to late 1800's, there was a big transformation in the Japanese Society when there was a transition from the old feudal samurai era into the modern era. With this transition, many changes occurred in the cultural identity and traditions, including martial arts. This shift considered that martial arts were no longer needed for actual warfare, instead many other art forms, focusing more on the historic and cultural significance than on practical proficiencies became more ritualized. Subsequently, a move in the 1930's to implement karate into the Japanese school system led to further changes in the methods and techniques as safety became a primary focus, along with discipline, mental focus and other benefits of Budo training. Contact was removed from karate competitions in the interest of safety and as a result, the techniques and strategies were modified to reflect that change.

Some styles even made further modifications by deciding that competitions were not necessary and placing greater emphasis on practicing techniques and forms. However, there were a few masters of the modern era who felt differently. For example, masters including Masutatsu Oyama, Founder of Kyokushin Karate and Kori Hisataka, Founder of Shorinjiryu Kenkokan Karatedo to name a few, felt that it was very important to keep the elements of contact in training and that competitions were also important for developing a robust skill set. They believed that the mental and spiritual gains that martial arts can develop needed to be built through testing oneself in realistic combat and realistic training. This was a similar idea to that of the old samurai, who developed the ability to keep a calm relaxed mind even when faced with mortal danger. These _Contact Karate_ styles have kept such ideas ingrained in their practice and continue to foster the ideology that competition is a very important key to building oneself as a martial artist. Professional trainers of these styles also believe that one must constantly test themselves against a variety of different and better opponents in a wide variety of settings so that one can evaluate their own strengths and weaknesses in order to constantly improve their skillset. Today, this is a main concept in Contact Karate. Furthermore, due to these differences in the various styles of martial art, one will find that the techniques, while similar to those taught in non-contact systems, have several fundamental differences related directly to the lack of contact in training and competitions in non-contact systems.

SHORINJIRYU KENKOKAN KARATEDO AND KOSHIKI KARATEDO

Out of the few full-contact styles of karate originating from Japan, Shorinjiryu Kenkokan Karatedo is one of the most scientifically developed and codified systems that has been shared around the world. On a fundamental level, this system emphasizes what is known as Bogu training, which involves the use of strong armored chest protectors to minimize the impact of powerful blows. This enables one to practice all the techniques with full contact on a real opponent, thereby being better able to develop strong precise contact. At the same time, one can also study the relationship of these techniques to movement, distancing, and timing. By learning powerful techniques in bogu training, one can develop the ability to take strong hits and minimize their impact while also gaining an appreciation for the range and distancing of different opponents. This "bogu" training and fighting is done with bare hands and feet which become stronger over time. The bone density in a trainee's hands and feet increases such that they can build powerful precise contact and strike hard surfaces safely and properly. On a technical level, this system emphasizes using the whole body when executing all techniques. To drive the power of the technique, one must engage in twisting, thrusting, or extension (depending on the technique) of the hips and shoulders being rooted by a lowered center of gravity. This system also emphasizes escaping motions over blocking, thereby allowing for faster counter techniques and different timing approaches.

Up until 1979, the bogu training in Shorinjiryu Kenkokan Karatedo was done using armor from the art of Kendo. This armor is a hard lacquered chest protector with a metal caged face guard. There is no doubt that this equipment has some limitations due to its hardness. In 1979, Hanshi masayuki Hisataka, son of the founder of Shorinjiryu kenkokan along with a team of engineers developed the "Supersafe Guard", a protective equipment, known as bogu using modern materials and technologies. The Supersafe Guard is a light weight chest guard reinforced by a plate of bullet-proof plastic at the core and a form fitting head guard with a bullet-proof plastic bubble that covers the entire face. This equipment allows for complete fluidity of movement and vision, enabling fighters to practice and fight using bare hands so that they can develop a fluid and powerful style of fighting and make effective use of their hands and feet as natural weapons without the need for padding.

With the birth of this new equipment, the Koshiki competition system was also born. This style is simply a competition system using the Supersafe Guard in a bare-handed fighting format. This method of training and fighting is of course standard in the Shorinjiryu Kenkokan system however, Koshiki as a competition system was created to serve as a testing ground for all styles. Hence, the World Koshiki Karate Federation was formed as the governing body of international Koshiki Karate. Today, World Koshiki Karate Championships are held annually and the best Koshiki fighters who practice all styles of martial arts from around the world attend to test themselves at the highest level of full contact karate. In recent decades, many Koshiki champions have moved on to professional fighting with outstanding success. A few notable Koshiki champions are Nathan "carnage" Corbett, an eleven-time world Muay Tai Champion, Alex Chambers currently in the UFC, Yoann Kongolo European K1 and kickboxing champion, Alexander Matmuratov Champion Russian MMA fighter, Masahito Hisataka undefeated MMA fighter in Japan, and many more who have graduated from the world Koshiki arena to a successful career in pro combat sports.

CHAPTER 1: DEVELOPING THE MIND, BODY, AND SPIRIT

1.1 WHY DOES ONE NEED TO KNOW HOW TO FIGHT? WHY TRAIN IN BUDO?

OVER THE YEARS, the focus of Karate training and Budo has changed due to many factors however, I believe that the original purpose of the practice of Budo and its training has remained relatively unchanged, although this purpose is not always fully understood by its practitioners. Budo means the martial way, it refers to the Japanese systems that were designed to guide the warriors of the day (known as samurai) and teach them the necessary skills to be honourable, courageous, and skillful in battle. These arts were ultimately designed to combine a warrior's mental and physical strengths in such a manner to unlock the warrior's full potential, thereby giving them their best chance for success. Ultimately, these warriors found that the most difficult opponent they had to face was themselves. They learnt that it is the mental and physical weaknesses within oneself that are ultimately responsible for one's own defeats and by mastering one's own weaknesses, one can ultimately be successful. This notion still holds true today for professional fighters, athletes, or anyone trying to be successful in life. Budo arts in their different forms attempt to impart a method or way of overcoming one's weaknesses and achieving one's full potential. It is this main idea or concept that has been at the center of the practice of Budo arts.

When looking at the idea of discovering one's full potential, there are many factors that must be considered. Of course, physical factors are one of them that I will discuss in more details in later chapters, but more importantly, there are also mental, emotional, and spiritual factors that are of great importance. In fact, the realities of the modern world present challenges and tough choices that require a person to be mentally strong and to have great determination in order to not only be successful but also be happy with the choices and efforts made. So how does a person develop this kind of "strong spirit" and overcome their fears, anxieties, anger, doubts, and other factors that are known to be detrimental in making good decisions? It is important to understand that some of these negative responses are caused by mental factors (i.e. those that are created in one's own minds like anger, self-doubt, fear etc) and by physiological factors that include the body's natural and uncontrolled responses to situations that are dangerous, highly stressful, or confrontational. These natural responses are the most difficult to overcome and gain control over as they require a person to face them directly in order to conquer them.

To effectively deal with difficult situations, one must face these challenges in a realistic manner to be able to properly replicate the body's natural responses. This is most important when dealing with fighting or defending oneself. Being able to control the body's responses when being struck or violently attacked by another individual is essential in any real-life fighting situation. For this reason, it is crucial that Budo arts be practiced under realistic conditions involving real contact, allowing a trainee to test the techniques and principals in realistic combat situations. In such training environments, one can overcome many of the body's natural responses, allowing them to effectively employ techniques and strategies rather than being crippled by one's own negative responses. In Karatedo, overcoming of these factors is referred to as the _development of the spirit_. A strong spirit is required for real fighting and defense as well as to effectively handle any difficult situation that may arise in life. Oftentimes, determination is the deciding factor in one's success or failure when attempting to accomplish or achieve a goal. Therefore, building a strong fighting spirit is essential to understanding and achieving one's true full potential.

In addition to the above-mentioned physiological factors, there are also several mental and, emotional, and spiritual factors that can pose as major obstacles in training, fighting, or other situations in life. Many of these mental, emotional and spiritual responses come from one's own ego and its response to one's interactions with others. An individual's feelings can be hurt and they can become angry or upset and have a variety of responses that can oftentimes cause them to make poor decisions based on subjective feelings rather than objective strategies and techniques. It is for this reason that humility and temperance are qualities that Karate and other Budo arts seek to develop in an individual. This is also the main reason for a strong emphasis on manner and etiquette in the dojo. By practicing a strong level of etiquette in the dojo such as by always remembering to bow and thank one's training partners and coaches, a trainee can develop a humble attitude and calm their ego over time. This can be highly beneficial for a trainee by allowing them to think calmly and make effective decisions even in emotionally stressful situations. In the Karate dojo, there is immense respect given to an instructor, also known as a sensei. It must also be noted that such respect is not intended for the instructor's benefit but rather it is for the student to develop a humble attitude that is not easily swayed by anger and emotion. Regardless of the style of martial art, it is important for all martial artists to develop their own ways to show respect and humility towards others because negative emotions in the dojo or gym can hinder learning and increase the chances of unwanted injuries. Ultimately, it is the instructor's or coach's responsibility to set the tone with respect to manner and etiquette in order to foster a positive training environment.

1.2 AN EFFECTIVE FORMULA FOR LEARNING

There is a concept that originates from old Japanese philosophical traditions known as _Shin Gi Tai_ and can be applied as a method for learning and developing martial arts techniques as well as to learn or develop other ideas or skills. The term _Shin Gi Tai_ literally translates to Mind (shin), Technique (gi), and Body (tai) such that it refers to an order or approach to learning or developing a skill. According to this philosophy, mental preparation is the key to success in learning and mastering a skill. Thinking about the technique or task at hand means to mentally understand what it will entail and to prepare the mind to engage oneself fully in the task. In this way, an individual can now look at the techniques objectively, thereby fully grasping the key points necessary for accomplishing the task. In the case of learning or developing fighting techniques, this phase may involve some physical practice but in a slower, lighter way so as to focus on the technical aspects of the techniques rather than power and speed. Lastly, the "tai" or body phase, the "shin" or mental phase, and the "gi" or technical phase come together in full physical practice, drawing on the knowledge and understanding gained in the first two phases to create and develop power, speed, timing, and other skills being practiced. By developing one's techniques and strategies using "shin gi tai", one will not only build and develop these techniques faster but will also gain a strong understanding of the concepts behind these techniques. By gaining a deeper understanding of the concepts rather than simply learning to copy or repeat a technique, one will be able to develop these techniques to a much higher level and be able to apply them in a variety of different situations. When one trains or practices these techniques, if one focuses directly on strong physical practice, they may end up missing or ignoring some of the important and finer points underlying these techniques and strategies. This may prevent one from truly developing their full potential. In other words, it is crucial for a marital artist to prepare mentally, to thoroughly study the techniques and strategies and to train on a regular basis!

Along with the idea of Shin Gi Tai, another important concept that originates from Japanese traditions is the idea of "_seeing through three eyes_". This refers to developing and having a strong understanding of three different perspectives. First, one's own perspective (1st eye) which refers to the way one views their surroundings and develops their own opinions, thoughts, and feelings. Second, the perspective of the person one is interacting with (2nd eye), including the other person's point of view, opinions, thoughts, and feelings. Third, an observer's perspective (3rd eye), who is objectively viewing the situation from the outside. In the case of a fighting situation, the 1st eye is the fighter's techniques, strategies, strengths, and weaknesses; the 2nd eye is the opponent's techniques, strategies, strengths, and weaknesses; and the 3rd eye is the referee's or judge's perspective as an outside observer of the fight. By studying and understanding these three perspectives when preparing for and competing in a fighting competition, a martial artist will be able to tailor their strategies to maximize their chances of success. At the same time, this concept can be beneficial in any situation that involves interaction with others because by understanding the perspectives of all those concerned, one will be more likely to make wiser and compassionate decisions.

1.3 BREATHING, TRAINING, AND FIGHTING

The development of proper breathing techniques for training and fighting is extremely important primarily because breathing is directly responsible for muscle fatigue and weakness. At the same time, when one attempts to apply force or strength, one's muscles require high levels of oxygen to perform at their full potential. On a basic level, one must develop what is referred to as abdominal breathing. This is where one uses the muscles of their diaphragm to push air into the lower parts of their lungs to pressurize it before exhalation. This kind of "abdominal breathing" creates a sort of back pressure that allows for more oxygen to be absorbed into the blood stream, thereby energizing the muscles and allowing for more powerful and explosive movements. Basic abdominal breathing can be achieved by deeply inhaling air through the nose, causing the abdomen and diaphragm muscles to tighten to create pressure on the air. Once the air is squeezed by the abdomen, it can be smoothly exhaled out through the mouth. Exhalation can be done at a fast or slow rate, depending on the task being performed. For example, when meditating or relaxing, exhalation would be slow and deliberate whereas, when fighting, exhalation should be fast and sharp, allowing for a faster intake of fresh air and maximum oxygen uptake.

During fights, when it comes to striking, it is important to understand how breathing affects one's ability to exert force and for one's muscles to recover from fatigue. The main concept to understand here is that one's ability to deliver force is maximized at the moment when one's lungs are full of air and that air is placed under pressure by the abdomen. A good example of this is how a weightlifter breaths when lifting heavy weights. The weightlifter inhales and holds that air in their lungs under pressure while initiating the lift and begins to exhale that air towards the end of the lift. This demonstrates that the weightlifter has the most strength when their lungs are full of air under pressure. The same concept can also be applied for striking. At the moment of contact with any strike, one should ideally have their lungs completely full of air and under pressure. In order to achieve this, one must first inhale just prior to execution of the technique such that the air is in a pressurized state at the moment of contact and then quickly exhale right after contact is made. In this way, one will be able to maximize their ability to deliver a powerful strike. For professional fighting that involve a lot of combination techniques, it is not possible to complete a full breath for each technique as there is not enough time in between combination of various techniques. To accomplish the same effect when executing fast combinations, a small amount of air can be forced out of the mouth through the teeth while each technique of the combination is delivered. These short exhales are very similar to how a person sneezes, where the abdomen contracts and a small amount of air is released through the teeth under high pressure. These short sneezes, just like exhales allow for a short inhale in between techniques, thus providing the muscles with a sufficient supply of oxygen during an extended combination. However, when throwing single power techniques, the breath can be held and tightened during the moment of contact to maximize power and exhaled immediately afterwards. However, it is important when performing combinations that the exhalation be done by pushing air out with the abdomen in a short pressurized manner such that the entire pressure in the abdomen is not released at once. If the pressure is fully released upon contact, a large amount of power will be lost, and the muscles will quickly become weak and fatigued. Therefore, it is essential to practice proper breathing when training for striking motions such that one can become accustomed to the optimal timing for coordination of the squeezing of the abdomen when executing all techniques.

1.4 LEARNING THE CONCEPT AND NOT ONLY THE TECHNIQUE

It is important to note that there is a difference between learning a technique and understanding the underlying concepts behind the technique. By understanding the concepts, before attempting to master the technique itself, one will be able to gain a much better understanding of how to train in that technique and improve their skillset through a variety of different drills and methods. In addition, by studying the concepts one will be able to identify opportunities to use them in different situations as will no longer be limited to a single technique that utilizes a given concept. The concepts behind fighting and fighting techniques are universal in the sense that they are applicable to more than just fighting. These concepts speak to the very foundation of human interactions and individual goals, fears, and anxieties. Therefore, by studying and understanding these principals, one can gain a better understanding of themselves and their interactions with others as well as have a better understanding of the techniques and the possibilities to apply them both inside and outside of the ring. A great example of this is discussed in the book "The art of war", written centuries ago by the warrior General Sun Tsu. These strategies of war have been applied with great success throughout time, by businessmen and professionals around the world in meetings and negotiations. In fact, in daily human interactions, it is the concepts behind these war strategies and not the techniques that are enabling people to be successful in their goals and ambitions. Likewise, when a person trains in Budo with the goal of understanding the concepts and their applications in addition to mastering the physical techniques, one can also gain a better understanding of the underlying concepts applicable to all aspects of life.

In this way, these concepts become practical in all stages of life, whether for younger or older individuals, and for martial artists facing their toughest opponent or a novice in the ring. A trainee must adapt their training throughout the course of life so as to have the techniques and abilities to face all of life's challenges using one's full potential. Many of the martial arts masters of the past serve as great examples of this as they remained strong and virile well into their 70's, 80's, and even 90's. It is my opinion that one's fighting abilities, both mental and physical become more important in one's later years in life rather than in one's youth. Hence, training in martial arts must be maintained as a way of life such that it is continued even after retiring from competitive fighting. However, modifications should be made to one's training regimen as one gets older to reduce focus on hard contact and increase training on fluid techniques to maintain one's strength and flexibility. In sum, one's greatest battle in life is the one an individual fights against themselves to overcome one's own problems and weaknesses. One must always be ready to fight, whether with an opponent, against an illness or injury, and against a myriad of challenges in order to successfully achieve one's goals in life.

CHAPTER 2: STANCES, POSTURES, MOVEMENTS, AND DISTANCING

ONE OF THE most misunderstood aspects of Karate and other forms of martial arts is the purpose and use of its several stances. Many people, including karate practitioners oftentimes view Karate stances as ritualized positions in which a person can stand in order to defend themselves. However, Karate stances were not intended to be used in this way but rather were intended as movements or positions used to execute specific techniques. These body positions, also referred to as stances were developed by observing natural human and animal movements as they performed their daily tasks such as lifting, pulling, pushing, running, jumping etc. For example, while executing the task of heavy lifting, one will automatically widen their stance and bend their knees in order to lift this heavy object effectively and prevent injury to one's body. This position is the same as a Karate horse stance or open defensive stance. Likewise, while pushing or pulling heavy objects, one would naturally utilize the front or forward stance (pushing) and the cat stance or back stance (pulling). Thus, while these stances are very important to understand and use in one's practice of martial arts, they are not meant for use as depicted in movies to show an impressive looking fighting position. In such mass media depictions, Karate stances are often confused with fighting postures and guards. However, these Karate stances are practical moveable positions that are tailored to tackle a specific opponent depending on their physical characteristics, techniques, and strategies. It is also important to understand the difference between these transitional stances and their uses, and the basic fighting stances or postures. The main purpose of the basic fighting stances or postures is to provide a balanced and mobile platform for the fighter to be able to execute their techniques and strategies, while the main purpose of the traditional stances is to aid in the execution of these techniques and strategies.

2.1 COMMON PRINCIPLES FOR STANCES AND POSTURES

While each stance or posture has its own distinct characteristics, there are some common foundation principles that all stances and postures share and are built on. These foundation principles are essential in building a solid base for all techniques and strategies. Firstly, one must understand the concept of the _body centerline_ and how it relates to the feet position. An easy way to understand this is by walking on a balance beam, whereby one's feet share the same line as the centerline of the body or the direction of one's path. From this exercise, a trainee can learn that it is difficult to keep their balance when their feet share this common line. A trainee can also learn this concept by simply standing on a flat surface where one's balance is much better when standing with their feet directly under the shoulders, at shoulder width apart in comparison to walking on a balance beam. From the concept of these two ideas, a trainee can form the foundation of all stances whereby, the set-up of all stances should start with the feet placed approximately at shoulder width apart, allowing the target line to cut directly through the stance with both feet on either side. This positions the target line going through the center of the body, allowing both sides of the body to defend and attack while keeping the opponent in the center. Figure 2.1 (below) illustrates the centerline and feet position to further demonstrate the body's position.

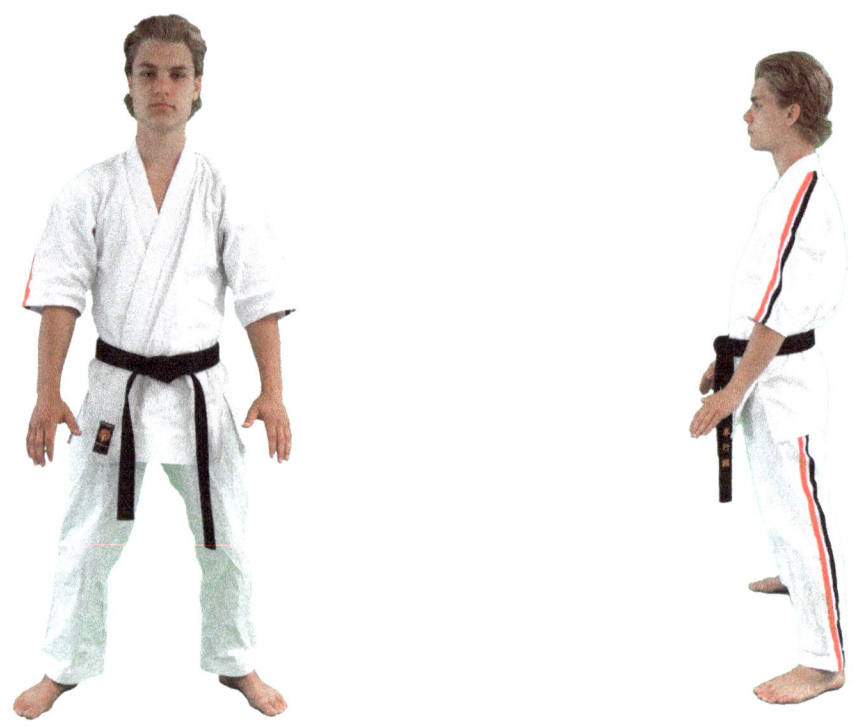

Figure 2.1: An illustration of the body's centerline and feet position.

Alternatively, some martial art styles recommend a fighting stance that is sideways to the opponent. However, for the purpose of contact fighting or real-life self-defense, this can be very dangerous as it exposes the individual's front leg to attack and provides a shortcut to their back where it is very difficult to defend oneself. At the same time, it limits the techniques that can be effectively used as the rear side of the body is not in an effective striking position, and the hips are not in a position to deliver power to the target.

Secondly, another very important foundation principle is that of the _center of gravity_, which refers to the positioning of one's body weight relative to the ground. The main idea is that when the center of gravity is positioned higher on one's body, it is easier to lose one's balance. Therefore, by lowering the body's center of gravity, one's body can become more stable and effectively heavier for the opponent to take down. Lowering the center of gravity can be achieved in two ways. First, the center of gravity can be lowered on one's body by simply bending the knees enough such that the body's main mass is lowered while still maintaining one's ability to move or react to external stimuli. Second, the body's center of gravity can be lowered by sufficiently relaxing the muscles in one's legs, neck, and shoulders to create the effect of "dead weight". When the body is rigid (i.e. muscles are tensed), they support a lot of the body's weight so that the weight is not all supported by the ground making it easier to be off balance. For instance, the effect is the same when trying to lift a sleeping person as they seem to be extra heavy because their body is not supporting any of the weight. Similarly, this principle should also be used in martial art stances by relaxing one's major support muscles just enough to create a dead weight-like effect. This will create a much more powerful stance which in turn will create more powerful techniques and allow an individual to absorb the force of an opponent's techniques more effectively, without being off balance or in a compromised position.

Lastly, an important principle for all stances is that of *posture*, which refers to the position of the back and torso relative to the ground. To maintain maximum stability and balance, the natural position for the torso is perpendicular to the ground. This allows the body's weight to be equally supported directly over the legs. By allowing the torso to tilt either forward or backward, the body's weight can be shifted away from over the legs and can result in a compromised balance. Good posture is extremely important when executing combination techniques. Tilting the body while executing a technique can throw a person out of position for the next technique, thereby rendering the combination either ineffective or cut short and leaving one off balanced and exposed. In other words, an individual must keep a straight back while performing all the stances and movements as it can affect one's ability to properly execute techniques and maintain balance.

2.2 TRADITIONAL STANCES

2.2.1 NATURAL STANCE (SHIZENTAI DACHI)

As the name implies, the natural stance known as Shizentai Dachi is basically the natural way a person would likely stand whereby their body is relaxed and balanced. It is similar to the way one would stand when having a conversation, with their feet at shoulder width apart, naturally supporting the weight of the body with a slight bend in the knees to allow for easy movements. In this position, one's arms are usually relaxed and remain towards the front of the body. It is very important to practice all techniques from this stance, particularly for real-life self-defense as it is the most common way to stand. Therefore, it is necessary to be able to effectively react to external stimuli from this position. This stance can be used from a full frontal alignment to one's opponent or at a 45 degree angle to one's opponent. Figure 2.2 (below) illustrates the body's position during this natural stance.

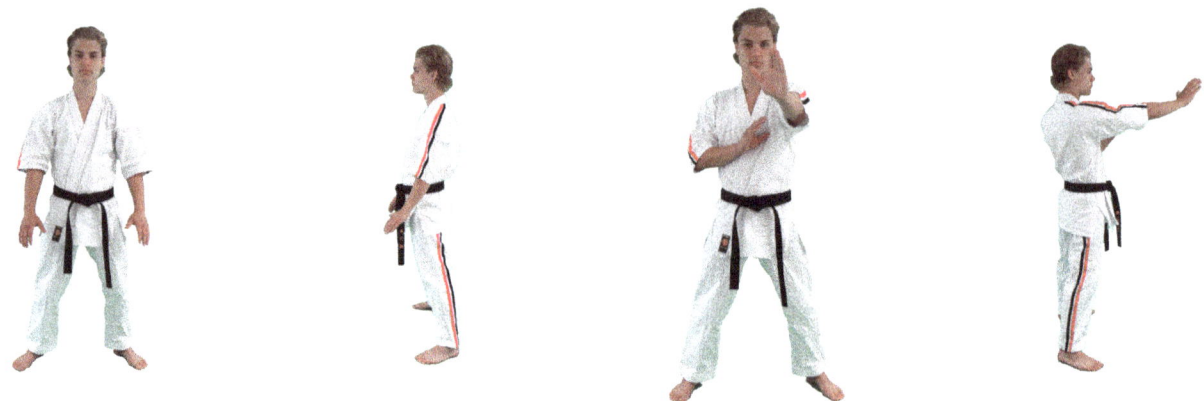

Figure 2.2: An illustration of the body's position during the natural stance, known as Shizentai Dachi.

2.2.2 FRONT STANCE (ZENKUTSU DACHI)

In this stance, the body's weight is shifted approximately 60% on the front leg, the feet are positioned at shoulder width apart and the stance is approximately 1½-2 shoulder widths in length. The hips and shoulders are predominantly facing forward and the heel of the back foot is on the ground. This stance is usually utilized at the moment of contact when delivering striking techniques with the hands. The shifting of the body's weight into this stance allows that weight to be added to the strike thus, making the strike more powerful. This stance is also utilized in grappling situations when one needs to push their opponent or to prevent themselves from being pushed backwards and also when executing certain throws. See Figure 2.3 (below) for a detailed illustration of the front stance.

Figure 2.3: An illustration of front stance, also known as Zenkutsu Dachi.

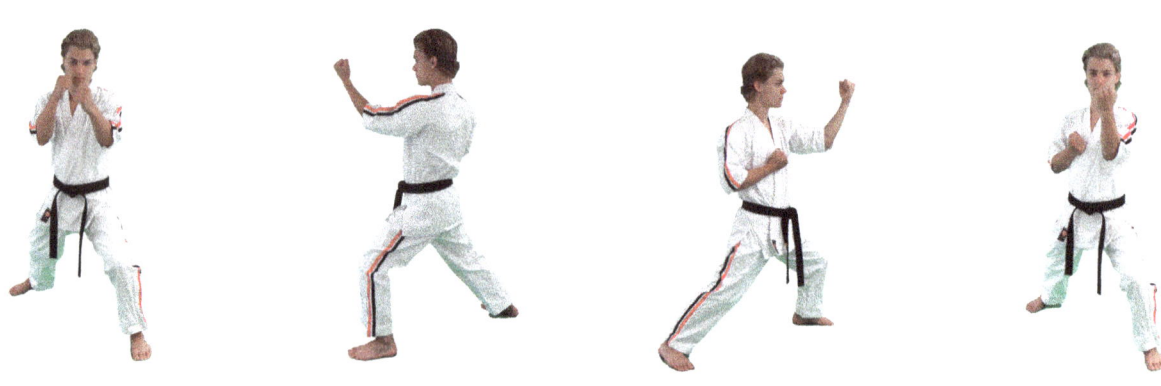

2.2.3 BACK STANCE (KOKUTSU DACHI)

In this stance, opposite to the front stance, the body's weight is shifted approximately 60% to the back leg with the feet at shoulder width apart and the stance at approximately 1½-2 shoulder widths in length. The hips and shoulders are slightly turned at a 45 degrees angle to the opponent. This stance is mainly utilized during escaping motions or defensive maneuvers. The shifting of the body weight to the back leg changes the position of the upper body moving the target from its original position and creating an escaping motion. The body weight is then loaded on the back leg allowing for a fast and powerful counterattack. This stance is also utilized in grappling situations when pulling one's opponent off balance or to execute a throw or sweep. Figure 2.4 (below) shows this stance in action.

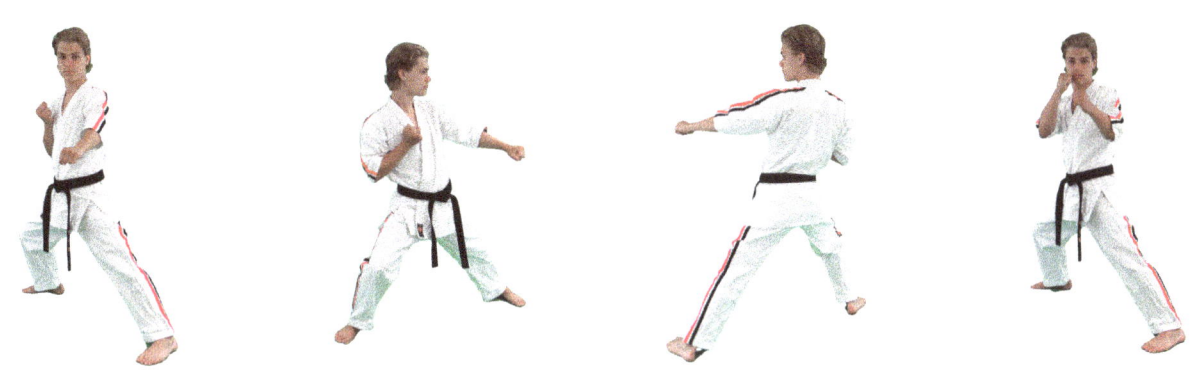

Figure 2.4: An illustration of the back stance, also known as Kokutsu Dachi in action.

2.2.4 CAT STANCE (NEKO ASHI DACHI)

In this stance similar to the back stance, approximately 70% of the body weight is shifted to the back foot while the front foot supports only 30% on the ball of the foot with the heel pointing up off the ground. The feet are positioned at shoulder width apart with the stance being one shoulder width in length. The back leg is slightly bent while the foot is turned outwards at an approximately 45 degrees angle. The hips and shoulders are at an approximate 30-45 degrees angle to the opponent. This stance is mainly utilized for explosive motions forward when attacking and also delivering kicking techniques with the front leg in a defensive position. Similar to the back stance, it can also be utilized in grappling situations when pulling an opponent and when executing certain foot sweeping techniques. See Figure 2.5 (below) for a detailed illustration of the cat stance.

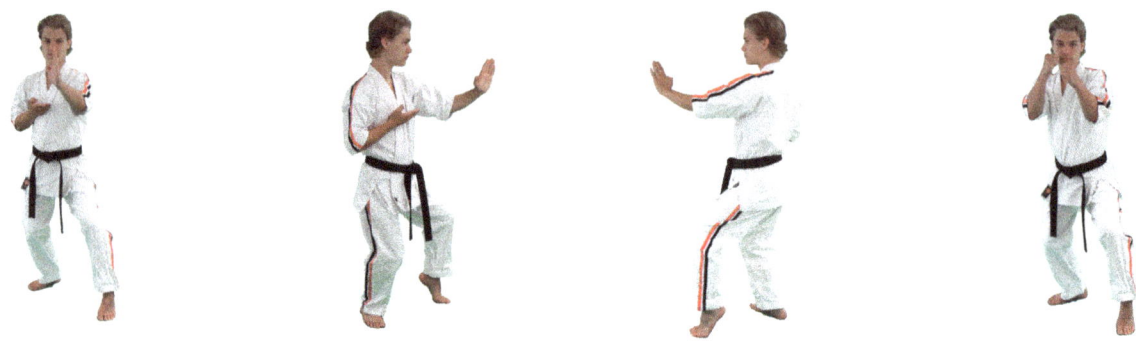

Figure 2.5: An illustration of the body's positioning during the cat stance (Neko Ashi Dachi).

2.2.5 CRANE STANCE (TSURU ASHI DACHI)

In many ways, the crane stance is opposite to the cat stance, whereby the weight is shifted approximately 70% to the front foot with 30% on the ball of the back foot and the heel pointing off the ground. The feet are shoulder width apart and the stance is also positioned at approximately one shoulder width in length. The front leg is slightly bent with the back leg extended behind. This stance is a very tall stance and maximizes the fighter's height and reach. It is one of the traditional stances that can also be used as a fighting posture. This strategy involves keeping distance between an opponent and oneself, thereby maximizing one's reach as would be the case when fighting against a shorter and more powerful opponent. This stance can be used when delivering striking techniques with the hands, executing them from a lowered position such as a fighting stance, using the raising of the body into this stance to generate more power during the execution of this technique. This stance can also be used in grappling situations when pushing and lifting one's opponent off balance and executing a throwing or sweeping technique. See Figure 2.6 (below) for a detailed illustration of the body's position during this stance.

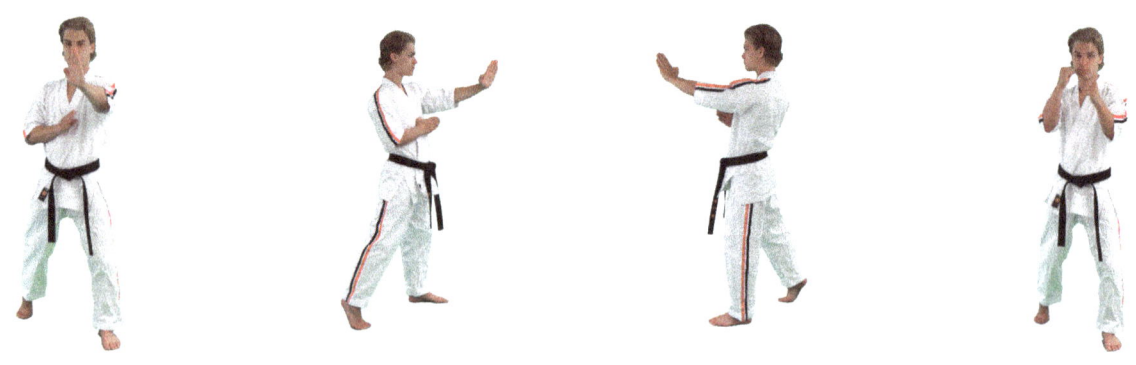

Figure 2.6: An illustration of the body's positioning during the crane stance (Tsuru Ashi Dachi).

2.2.6 OPEN DEFENSIVE STANCE (SOTOBIRAKI JIGO HONTAI DACHI)

This stance is similar to the horse stance that is prevalent in most karate styles. It does not assume a sideways posture to the target, but rather a centered position on the target line to the opponent, similar to the other stances described in this book. The feet must be kept at shoulder width, with the stance being 1½-2 shoulder widths in length. The body weight must be equally distributed over both feet and the knees must be turned outwards and bent at an approximately 30-40 degrees angle. The hips and shoulders must be positioned at approximately 45 degrees to the opponent. This is a very stable and rooted stance and is also one that can be used as a favorable fighting posture where the strategy is to hold one's ground when attacked. This stance can also be used in grappling situations to root the body, thereby providing a strong base to defend certain throws and takedowns. It is also utilized when lifting the opponent's body from a lowered position and when striking down to the ground from a standing position. See Figure 2.7 below for details.

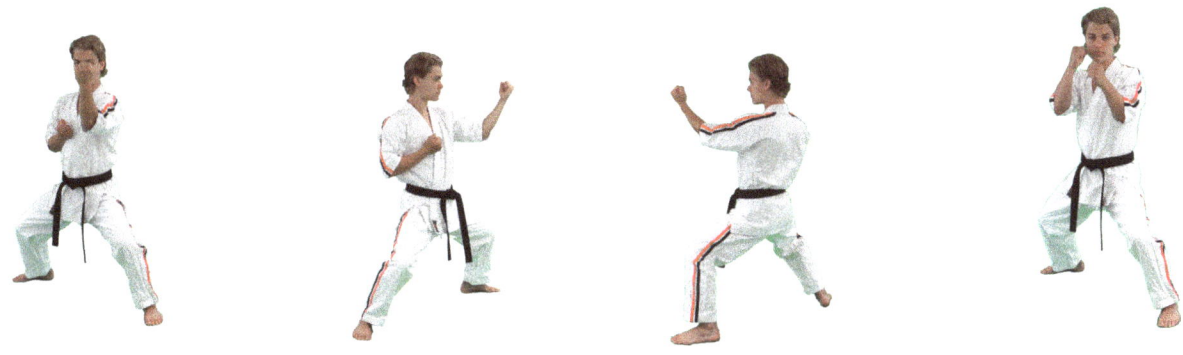

Figure 2.7: Front and side views of the Open Defensive Stance (Sotobiraki Jigo Hontai Dachi).

2.2.7 THE FIGHTING STANCE (FIGHTING POSTURE)

As previously mentioned in this chapter, the fighting stance or posture is the position that a fighter stands in when engaged in a fight, prior to execution of a fighting technique. In other words, it refers to how the fighter stands in between exchanges, when the fighter is moving around and looking for an opening to attack or waiting for an attack to happen. As such, this stance must be stable, mobile, and allow the fighter to execute techniques from both left and right sides of the body. At the same time, it must provide protection or cover to the center line of the body which is where many of the body's vitals are located (i.e. face, throat, solar plexus, and groin). During this stance, the feet must be positioned shoulder width apart with the stance being 1½-2 shoulder widths in length and the weight evenly distributed on both feet with the heels just lifting off the floor so that the weight is on the balls of the feet and the heels are almost touching the ground. The knee of the front leg should be bent at an approximately 30 degrees angle and the foot turned slightly inward providing some cover for the groin and assisting in defensive motions. The back leg must be extended behind and also slightly bent with the foot turned slightly outward and the knee turned slightly inward. The hips and shoulders must be slightly turned at an approximately 30-45 degrees angle also providing some cover to the body's vitals. The arms should be kept relaxed with the elbows kept in and pointing downwards. The lead hand must be slightly in front of the face in the body's center line at approximately eye level and the back hand slightly in front of the shoulder or towards the center of the body at approximately the height of the jaw line or solar plexus. The way in which a fighter positions their guard will depend on the fighting they are engaged in. The ways in which a fighter positions their hands in a fighting stance will depend on whether a fighter is using boxing gloves, MMA gloves, or no gloves as in the case of Koshiki fighting, or whether grabbing, throwing, and submission techniques are allowed. See Figure 2.8 for details on the fighting stance and variations of guard positions.

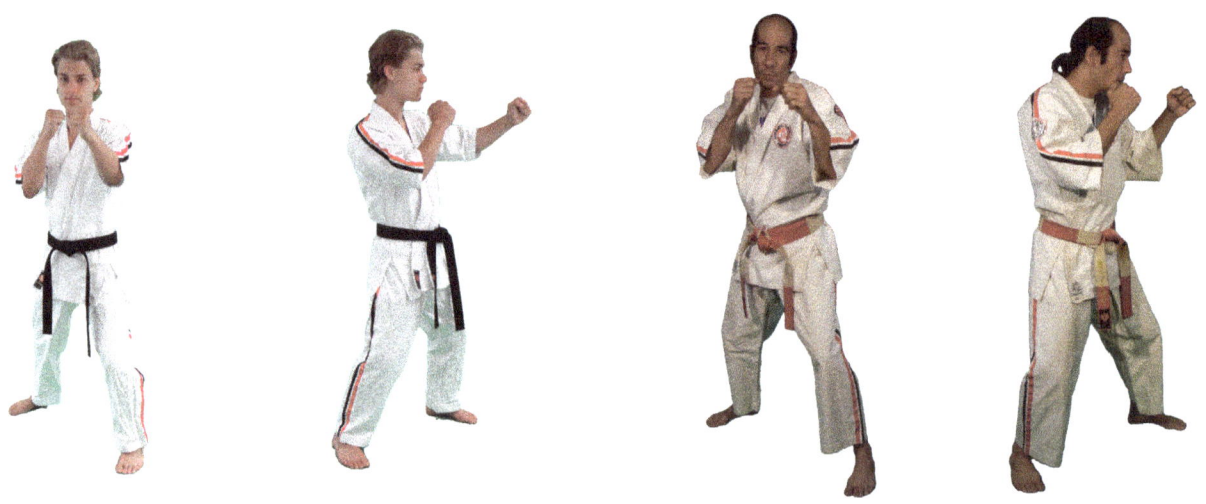

Figure 2.8: Illustrations of the fighting stance, posture and guard positions

2.3 DISTANCING AND MOVEMENT

2.3.1 DISTANCING

One of the first and most important points that must be understood when facing any opponent is how far away the target is and how to cover that distance in the most effective way. For this purpose, there are 3 main distances that must be identified, referred to as close distance (Chikama), middle distance (Chuma), and long distance (Toma). Close distance is the distance at which both fighters can touch each other's guard without stepping. In this way, either fighter can make contact with their target with only a small step. Middle distance refers to the distance at which both fighters are just unable to reach out and touch hands with each other, however if they lean slightly forward, they can touch each other. It is the most common fighting distance. Lastly, long distance refers to the distance at which both fighters even when reaching and leaning in cannot touch hands. See Figure 2.9 below for illustrations of these three distances.

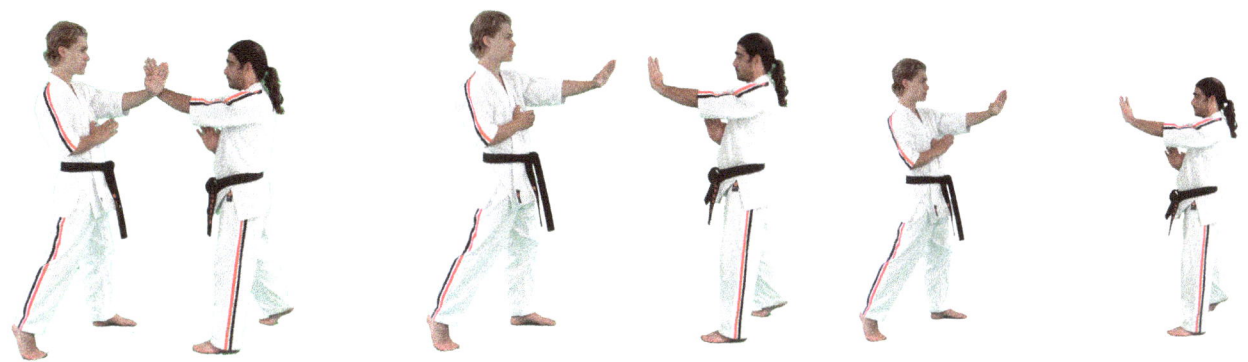

Figure 2.9: Illustrations of the three main distances in a fighting stance: Close distance (Chikama), Middle distance (Chuma), and Long distance (Toma).

2.3.2 MOVEMENT

A fight is not a stationary activity, rather it is a dynamic activity that requires constant motion. Fighters are constantly moving to find an opening to attack or to avoid an attack. At the same time, one's opponent is seldom standing close enough to attack from a stationary position requiring movement to make contact. Movement therefore is one of the most important aspects of fighting and can make a difference between success and failure in the ring. It is important to understand and practice all types of movements that relate to fighting so that over time one's movements become explosive and efficient.

There are three types of movements related to fighting, namely offensive movement, defensive movement, and positioning movement. First, offensive movement refers to how a fighter must step and move when attacking. Second, defensive movement refers to how a fighter must step and move while escaping and avoiding one's opponent. Lastly, positioning movement refers to how a fighter should step and move when looking for an attack opportunity or waiting to counterattack. The type of step that must be used in any of these situations should be determined by the distancing involved. It is also important to understand what step(s) should be used based on distance that must be covered.

2.3.3 TYPES OF STEPS

There are three steps that can be used either offensively or defensively when fighting to effectively cover distance between oneself and the opponent. These steps include the cat step, the sliding step, and the lunging step (forward and reverse). In addition, there is also a fourth step which utilizes the previous three steps, known as the Zig Zag step or lightning step (Denko Ashi).

A. Cat Step (Neko Ashi)

Firstly, the Cat Step (Neko Ashi) involves pushing off the back leg and stepping forward with the front leg when attacking as well as pushing off the front leg and stepping backwards with the back leg when escaping or moving away. This is a quick and explosive step but is limited as to how much distance can be covered and is thus recommended for use when attacking and defending from a close distance position. See Figures 2.10 and 2.11 (below) and the accompanying video for illustrations of the cat step.

CAT STEP: SIDE VIEW

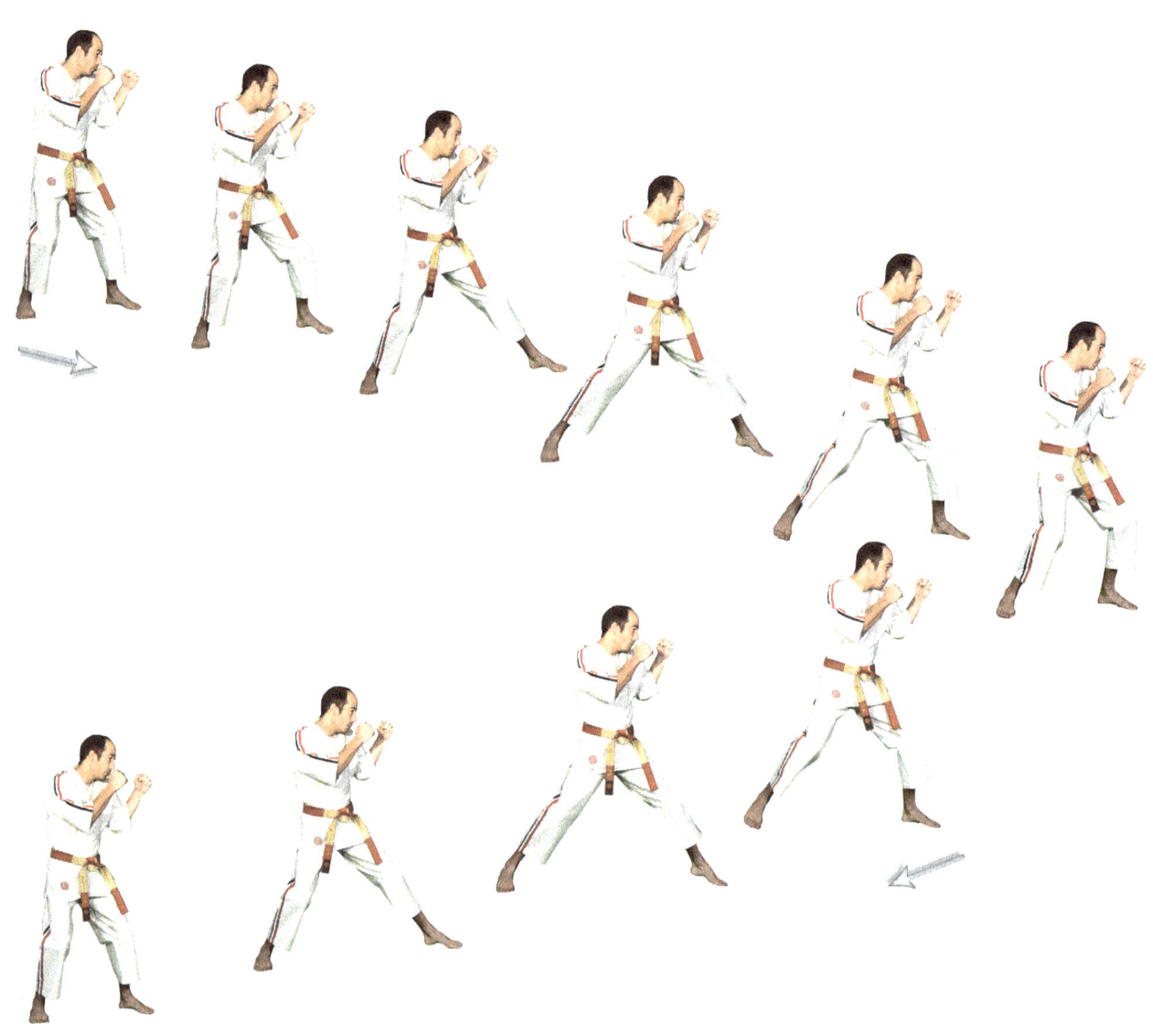

Figure 2.10: Illustrations of the cat step, side view.

CAT STEP: FRONT VIEW

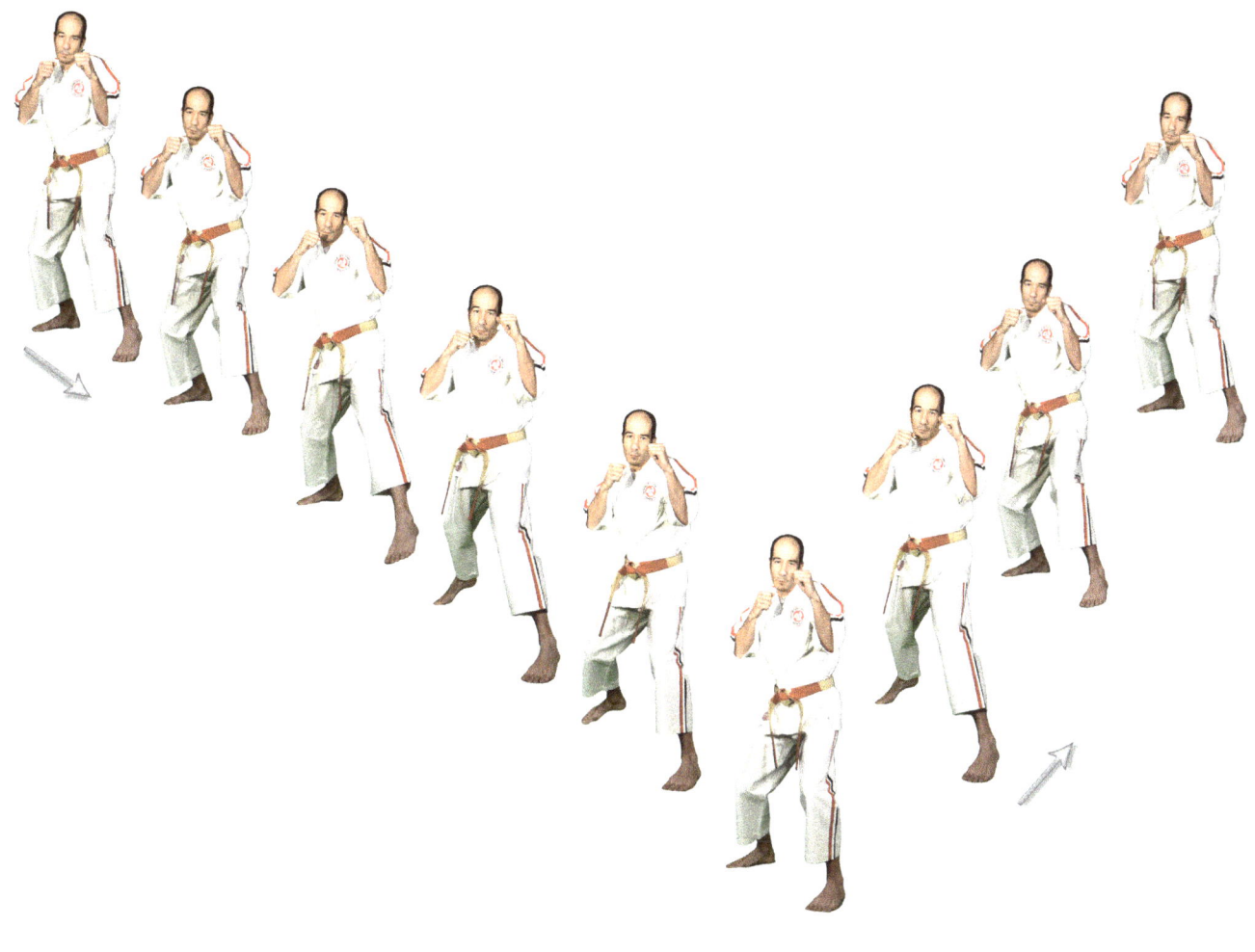

Figure 2.11: Illustrations of the cat step, front view.

B. Sliding Step (Okuri Ashi)

Secondly, the sliding step (Okuri Ashi) can be used when attacking, whereby the back foot must be slid forward towards the target and then pushed off the ground, in a similar way as the cat step. When escaping or moving away from the opponent, the front foot must first be slid backwards and then pushed off the ground, stepping back with the back foot as in the cat step. The additional step with the back foot prior to stepping with the front foot increases the amount of distance that can be covered and therefore is recommended for use when attacking and defending from a middle distance position. See Figure 2.12 below and the accompanying video for illustration of the sliding step.

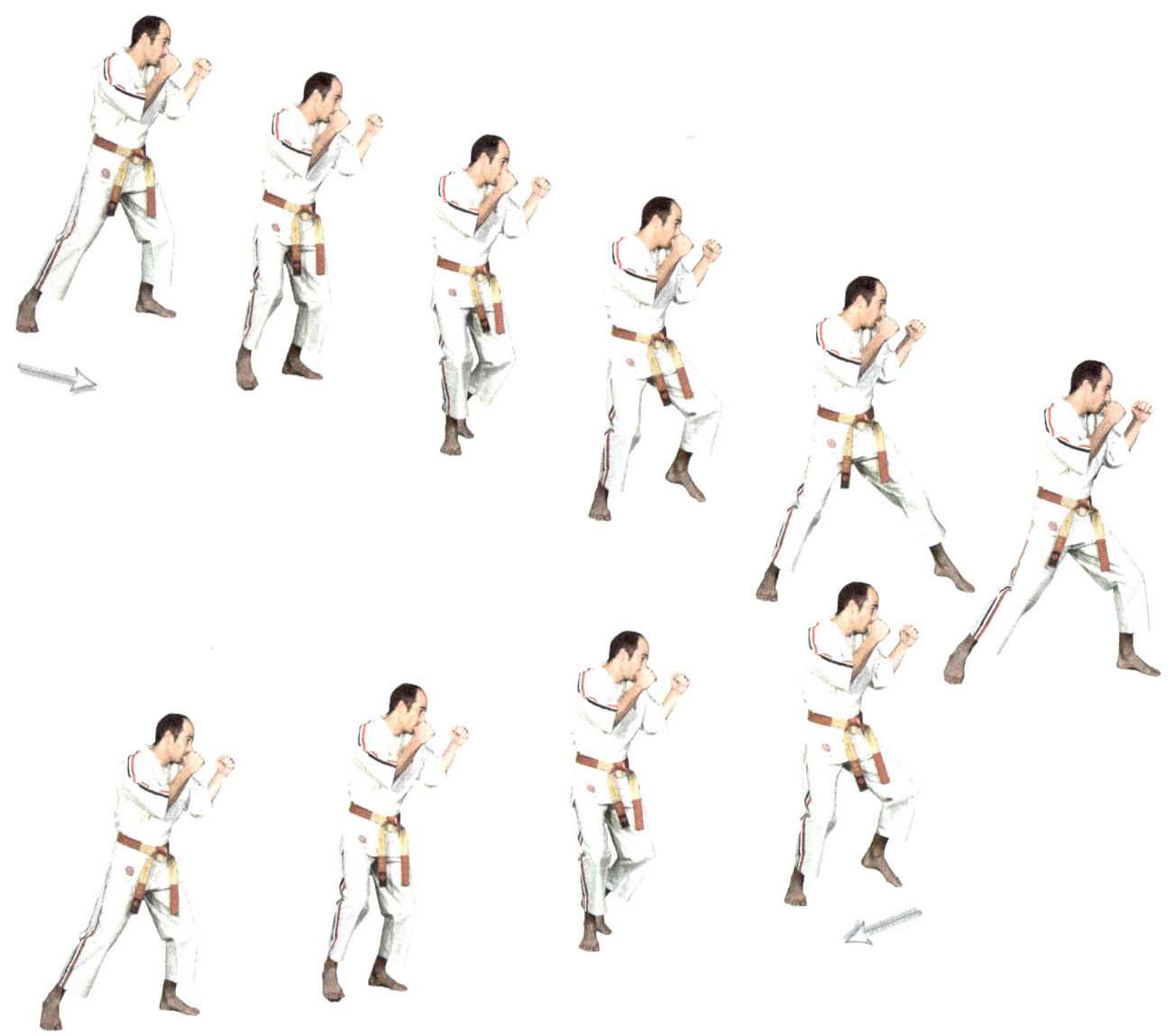

Figure 2.12: Illustrations of the sliding step.

C. Lunging Step (Oi Ashi)

Thirdly, the lunging step (Oi Ashi) can be used when attacking one's opponent. During this step, the back foot must step towards the target and become the front foot, effectively switching one's stance. When escaping or moving away, the front foot must step backward and become the back foot. This switching of stance as one steps forward covers the largest amount of distance and is therefore recommended for use when starting from a long distance or when creating space from one's opponent defensively. It is important to keep the center line of one's body facing the target throughout this entire step as excessive turning of the upper body during the lunging step will slow down the motion and also expose oneself to an attack while in mid-step. It is also important to note that when passing the front leg and stepping forward, the back leg should pass through the center of one's stance and then back out to the shoulder width apart position. By making the entire movement along the shoulder width line, the step becomes slower and off balanced and exposes the body's center line to an attack while in mid-step. See Figures 2.13 and 2.14 below and the accompanying video for an illustration of lunging step.

LUNGING STEP: FRONT VIEW

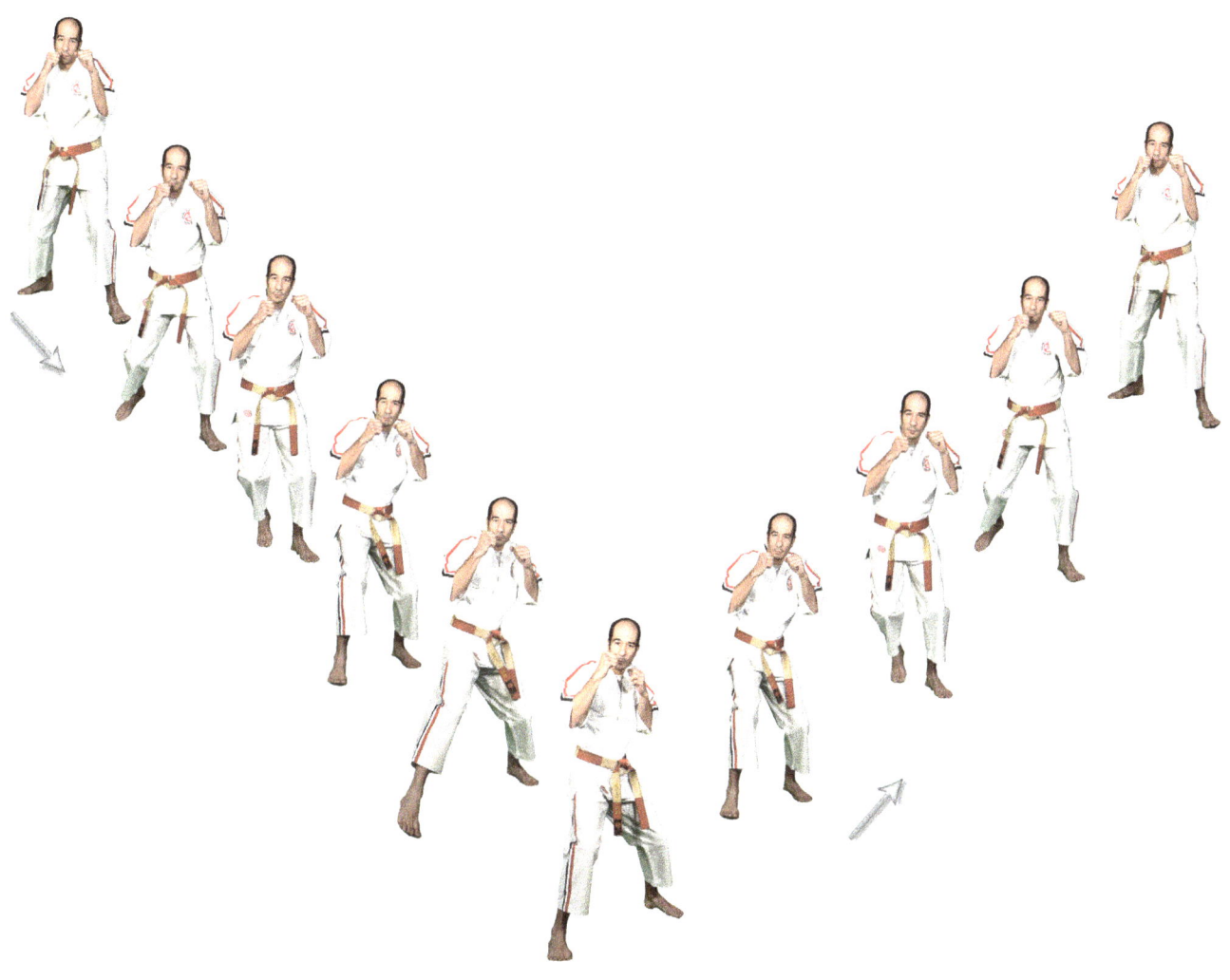

Figure 2.13: Illustrations of the lunging step from the front view.

LUNGING STEP: SIDE VIEW

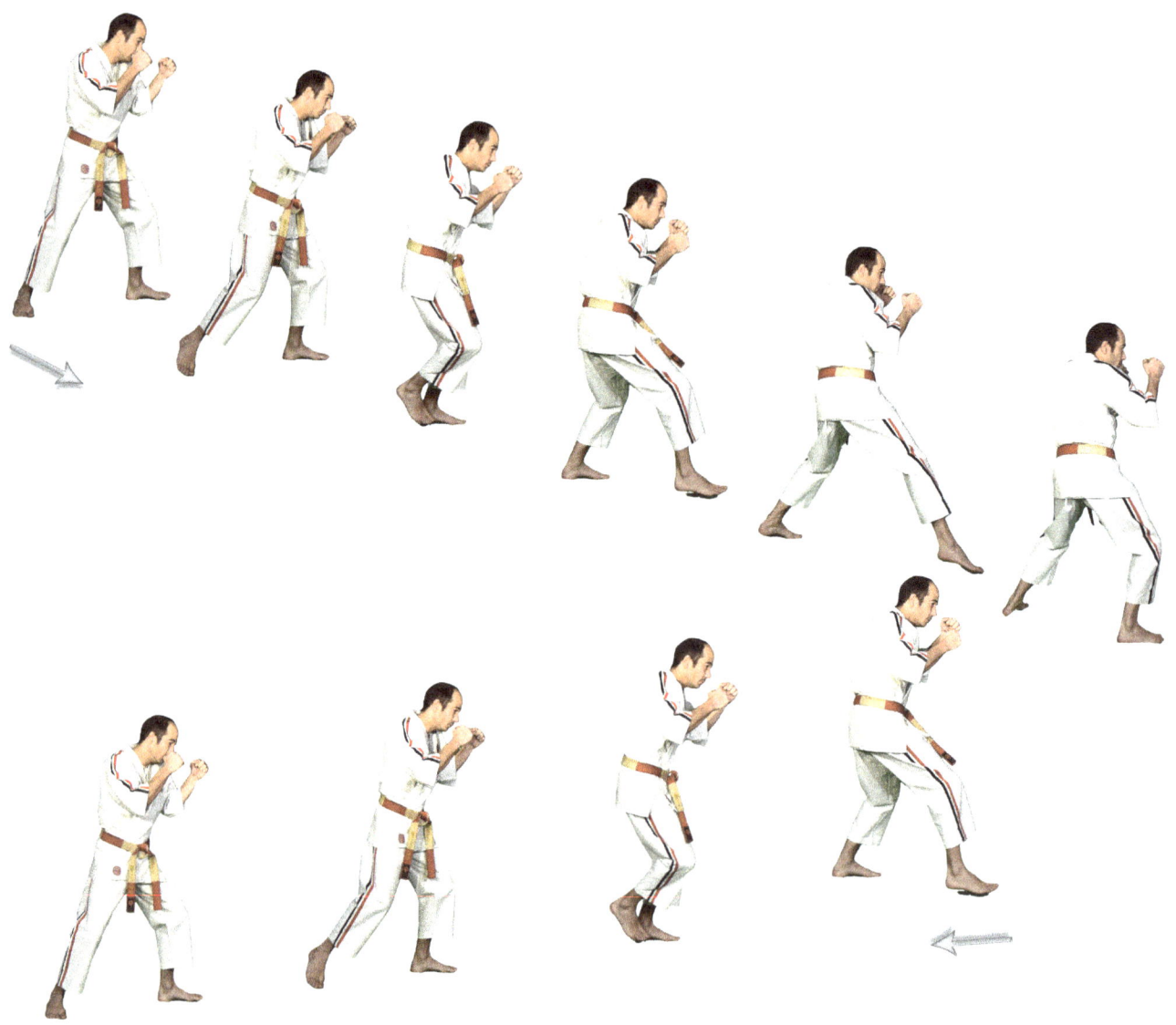

Figure 2.14: Illustrations of the lunging step from the side view.

D. Reverse Lunging Step (Ushiro Oi Ashi)

Another form of the lunging step is the back/reverse lunging step (Ushiro Oi Ashi), also known as a turning back step. It is the reverse of the lunging step described above. This step is performed by turning the body backwards and stepping forward with the back foot until it becomes the front foot. It is mainly used during the execution of spinning techniques such as the spinning back fist or spinning back elbow but can also be used to cut off an opponent's movement and create an opening for attack. To perform this step, one must begin by stepping across the centerline with their front foot. Then, one must quickly rotate their head and body backwards until they are facing the target. This must be followed by a step through the center line and out towards the target adopting the opposite fighting stance to the one executed at the start and properly centering oneself to the target. When used in a defensive manner, the front foot must be moved backwards and across the center line creating space, then the back foot must take over and move to the target to effectively execute this technique. See Figures 2.15 and 2.16 (below) and accompanying video for illustration of back/reverse lunging step.

REVERSE LUNGING STEP: FRONT VIEW

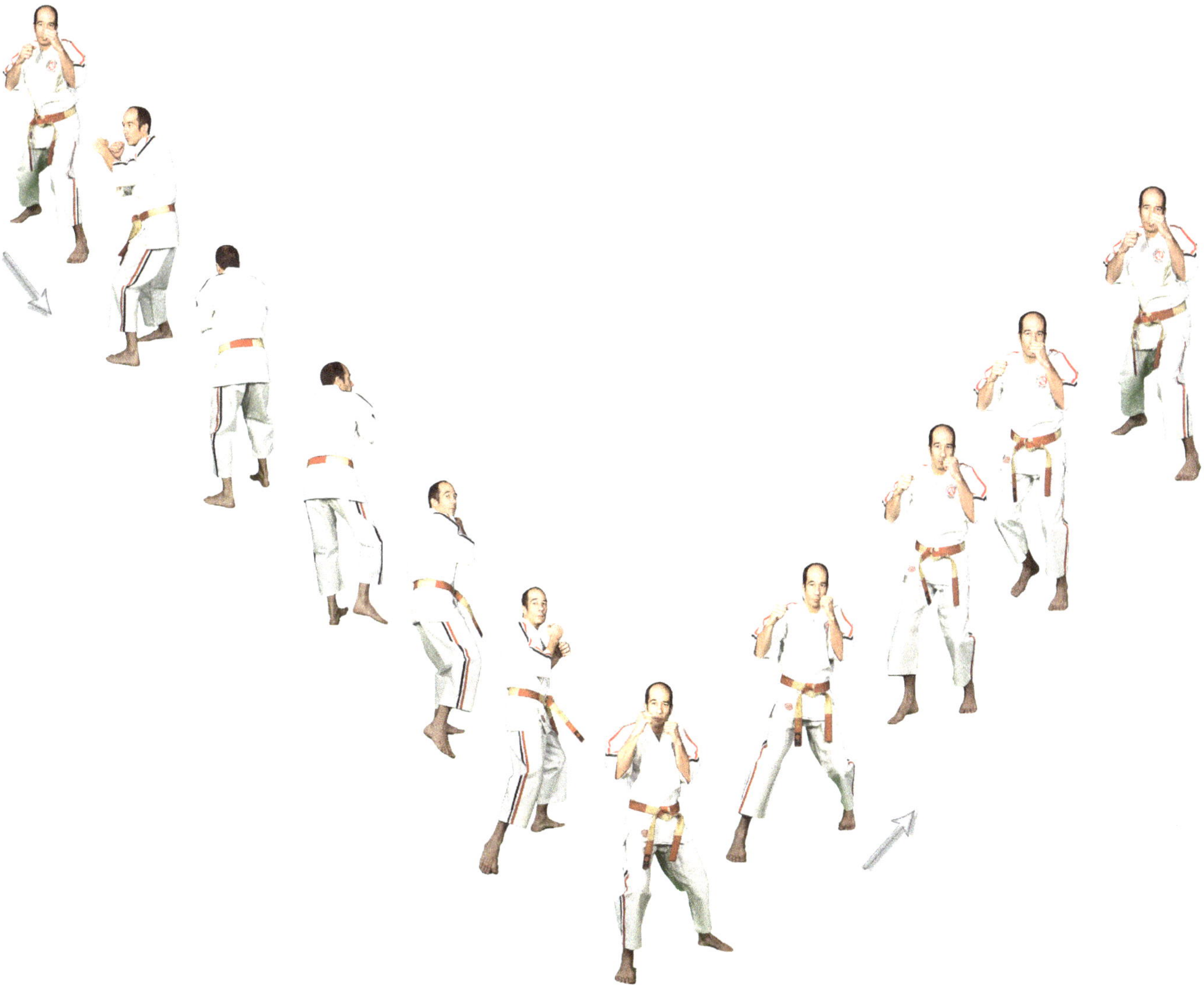

Figure 2.15: Illustrations of the reverse lunging step from the front view.

REVERSE LUNGING STEP: SIDE VIEW

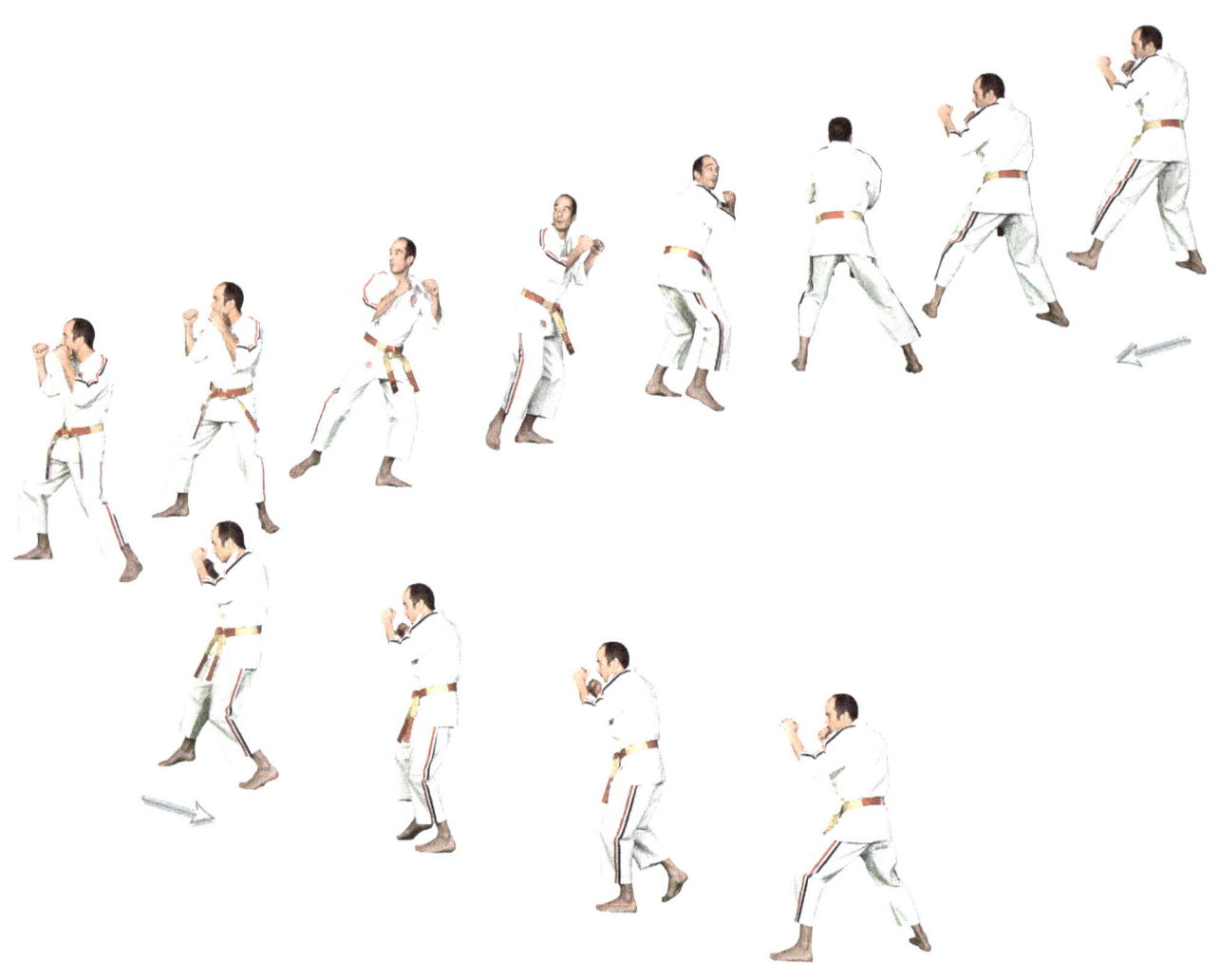

Figure 2.16: Illustrations of the reverse lunging step from the side view.

E. Zig Zag Step (Denko Ashi)

There is also a fourth step which utilizes the previous three steps, it is called the Zig Zag step or lightning step (Denko Ashi). This step is used for quickly changing angles and direction of movement either offensively or defensively. As the name implies, the pattern of this movement forms the shape of a lightning bolt and has a zig zag effect. It is executed by using any of the above-mentioned steps or a combination of them. First, this step can be used to move to a position approximately 45 degrees off the target line and then approximately 45 degrees to the opposite angle with the following step. This 45 degrees angle can be increased or decreased depending on various factors such as height, reach, and weight difference of the opponent. The use of this movement can be very effective especially in defensive motions because changing directions like this can make it difficult for the opponent to sustain a prolonged attack. It can also be effective when attacking as it can allow one to attack while staying off the opponent's center line or attack line, thereby cutting down on the techniques one's opponent can use for counterattack. See video for demonstration of the lightning step.

2.3.4 POSITIONING MOVEMENTS

Positioning movements refer to the movements used when one is not engaged with the opponent. These movements usually involve either circling the opponent or moving in and out of range in order to create an attack opportunity or to entice the opponent to attack. Circling one's opponent to create an opportunity is a very commonly used method in many types of contact fighting. It is particularly effective as it allows one to keep changing the target line, making it harder for the opponent to attack and can create moments when the opponent may not be ready to defend against one's attack.

Circling the opponent can be done either by circling to the back side or circling to the front side. In the case of a left stance, one's back side is in a clockwise direction to the opponent and the front side is in the counter-clockwise direction to the opponent. Circling to the back side can be done by stepping sideways with the front foot and having the back foot follow afterwards by pivoting one's body so as to keep the centerline focused on the opponent and returning back to a solid fighting stance.

Repeating this movement over and over creates the effect of circling around one's opponent. Circling to the front side is done by stepping to the side with the back foot and having the front foot follow afterwards while also remaining centered to the opponent and returning back to a solid fighting stance.

Repeating this step will circle one counter-clockwise around the opponent. It is very important NOT to circle to one's back side by leading with the back foot instead of the front foot. The same applies for circling to the front side and leading with the front foot instead of the back foot. By doing this, with every step, one will be crossing one foot either in front or behind the next foot, leaving one with a moment with one's legs crossed and unable to defend an attack which can be very dangerous in a real contact fight. Another important note about circling is that one must pay close attention not to allow the distance from the opponent to increase or decrease without the intention of doing so. If a fighter fails to take note of any changes in distance with the opponent, they may be unexpectedly attacked and will not be able to effectively defend oneself.

Another method of using movement to create an opportunity is by moving in and out of the opponent's range. This is done by pushing off the back foot and moving forward with the front foot and entering the outer edge of the opponent's range. Then, pushing off the front foot and moving the back foot to its starting position. These in and out movements should be fast and explosive so as to give a brief moment to assess the opponent's reaction. If a fighter enters the opponent's range and they don't react or react slowly, one would have an opportunity to attack. Likewise, if one favors counterattacking, one can use this method to bait the opponent into making an attack, thus creating an opportunity to counterattack.

2.3.5 BUILDING FOOTWORK AND MOVEMENT

Building strong fast footwork and movement is important for all fighters. Sufficient amount of time must be spent improving one's footwork and explosiveness. One must practice all of the different stepping motions focusing on speed and explosiveness while paying close attention to maintaining good balance throughout all movements. Resistance bands can also be used when practicing all movements to improve speed and explosiveness. Another way of practicing and improving footwork is to have a partner attack with striking techniques while one uses only movements to avoid, at the same time being aware of opportunities for counterattack.

It is also very important to train in all striking techniques with the different stepping motions, getting used to the changes in timing and the slight differences in delivering the techniques with the different steps and covering the different distances. This will help to build one's ability to select the best movement for covering the necessary distance and sync that movement with the execution of one's techniques.

Practicing all techniques with a partner and working through the different distances and steps both offensively and defensively is highly recommended and will help one to develop strong skills for moving and striking and combining the two. Refer to the accompanying video for methods on building footwork and movement.

CHAPTER 3: PUNCHING, KICKING, AND STRIKING

REGARDLESS OF THE martial arts style or fighting competition, it is the goal of most fighting martial artists to maximize the amount of force that they can generate and deliver to their opponent. Being able to hit harder is always a benefit to any fighter and in order to achieve this, one must understand all the factors that contribute to generating power or force in the different punching, kicking, and striking techniques. Based on Newton's Laws of Motion, it is well understood that Force = Mass x Acceleration. How does this apply to kicks and punches in the practice of martial arts? This means that the amount of force one can deliver is equal to the amount of one's body weight exerted upon the opponent during this technique multiplied by the rate of change in speed, also known as acceleration that a fighter travels at, from a stationary position to the point of impact with the opponent. In other words, the greater the amount of body weight exerted during this technique, the greater the amount of force generated. At the same time, the higher the acceleration, the greater the amount of force generated. With an understanding of this principle, one can then look at both mass and acceleration as two factors that can be maximized to develop maximum force in any punch, kick, or strike.

How can a fighter exert more mass into their techniques? The answer to this lies in several factors, some of which are specific to each technique. Nonetheless, the general idea is the same regardless of the technique, whereby a fighter must use the large mass of their body to generate momentum for the technique and also align the body so that it can drive that momentum into the target. This can be accomplished by either twisting the hips and shoulders, thrusting the hips forward, rotating the body in a circular motion or raising or lowering the body depending on the technique being executed. It is also important to understand that the ability to twist, thrust, or rotate the hips and shoulders can be affected by the position of the feet. It is therefore important to know and understand the different feet positions for the execution of the different striking techniques so as to allow for a full extension and/or rotation of the hips and shoulders thus, maximizing the amount of body weight driving the technique. Feet position will also affect one's ability to support the momentum generated by the hips and shoulders and drive it through the target. The optimal hip and body movements and feet positions will be discussed for each technique later in this chapter.

There are many factors involved in maximizing acceleration. Of course, there are many exercises that can help condition the muscles to be more explosive and somewhat faster. However, for the purpose of this book, I will focus on the techniques involved in generating speed and making fighting techniques faster. The main concept in generating speed is the same principle used in most sports or activities involving striking of any object such as in baseball, golf, volleyball, tennis, and many other physical sports. Tense muscles move slowly than relaxed ones. Therefore, to generate speed, one must generate momentum with mass of their body and allow their hands and feet to remain as relaxed as possible until the point of contact when the muscles must tighten and harden to drive the impact. The tension is then immediately released and muscles are relaxed after impact. This form of movement creates a kind of whipping effect that generates immense speed driven by weight. For this purpose, it is important to train in all techniques with the focus on relaxing the striking weapon and initiating the technique with the core muscles whipping the technique out to the target. It is also important to practice timing the tightening of the muscles of the weapon (i.e. fist or foot) at the exact moment of contact which helps to maximize impact and stabilize the joints of the arm or leg that one is striking with.

Along with mass and acceleration, another important factor that can affect the power of a technique is the positioning of the contact point in relation to the maximum extension of the technique. In other words, is the contact point at the end of the technique? Or is the contact point just before the end of the technique? To maximize force delivered to the target, the contact point should be positioned a little short of the maximum extension of the technique. This will allow the technique to penetrate the target and the force to be delivered completely rather than being stopped at the surface. By using the hips and shoulders to drive the technique through the target in this way and using good relaxed delivery and timing, a trainee can develop extremely fast and powerful penetrating techniques.

3.1 COMMON MECHANICS FOR STRIKING TECHNIQUES

One of the most important concepts to develop for one's striking techniques is the Japanese concept of "Ashi Sabaki, Tai Sabaki, Gi Sabaki", which translates to "foot work, body work, technique work". Simply put, this refers to the mechanical order in which to execute any technique. In this way, when executing a technique, first the feet must move into the correct position (footwork), then the twisting or thrusting of the hips and shoulders (body work), and finally followed by the release of the technique itself. In doing this, the momentum will be built from the ground, move through the body and explode like a whip out to the end of the technique. It must be noted that this concept must be built into the technique and performed as one fluid motion, whereby each part flows into the next. See illustration of this concept in attached video.

Another concept that works alongside the above-mentioned concept and is also very important for the development of high level techniques is, "stomping step, body drop, hip extension", also known as "Fumikomi Ashi, Otoshi Mi, Hineri Goshi" in Japanese. This concept represents the mechanical order for positioning the body weight to maximize its delivery into the target. In this way, when executing a technique, first the footwork must be done with a stomping action so as to create some momentum rising up through the leg into the torso (fumikomi ashi). Then, simultaneously the body weight must be dropped by flexing the knees, which positions the body weight to be driven by the leg muscles (Otoshi mi). Lastly, the hips and shoulders must be twisted or thrusted initiating the execution of the technique. By developing techniques that follow this order, a trainee can maximize the weight exerted into the target by using the legs to support and drive the twisting or thrusting of the hips when executing these techniques. As in the above-mentioned concept, this concept must also be built into one smooth, fluid motion and not performed as three separate motions. See demonstration of this technique in the attached video.

3.2 CONTACT, PRECISION, AND BOGU TRAINING

In order to have a full understanding of any technique, a martial artist must properly understand the concept of that technique both in theory and in practice. In other words, it is not enough to practice techniques in the air, they must also be practiced with real contact so as to fully understand the best way to use the mechanics of the technique in order to deliver maximum contact to the target. Therefore, it can be understood that the motions involved in the technique and making contact with the opponent during the execution of the technique are two distinct concepts. It is important to understand that every technique has an end point or a point of maximum extension. Proper contact can be made when the maximum extension of the technique is placed just before the target and the technique is tightened as it reaches its extension, making contact with a precise part of the weapon (fist or foot). This kind of precise contact can be developed over time through contact practice focusing on good timing, extension, and focus. Developing precise contact is best done through training with bare hands and feet.

Training with padded hands and feet may not be as effective because precision is not required to avoid injury when a mistake in contact is made using padded hands and feet. In other words, when wearing wraps and gloves, a trainee can get away with many mistakes in contact, that if made while bare handed would result in injury to the hands. When striking bare handed, one must be very precise and therefore, develop both power and precision at the same time. For this purpose, one of the best training methods is the use of Bogu (protective armor) as a way of practicing contact techniques on an actual opponent. This idea of using protective armor to train for fighting techniques is a very old idea that is passed down from the feudal days of Japan when the samurai trained for actual combat. In modern times, the same idea has been used in many martial art styles where there is a need for real contact to be made. For example, the art of Kendo has used Bogu since its beginning in samurai swordplay and there are also a few other karate styles that have emphasized this kind of training. The main one is Shorinjiryu Kenkokan Karatedo which in 1979 developed the Koshiki competition system to utilize the idea of Bogu in a bare hand contact fighting competition and the supersafe protective gear was invented for this purpose. See Figure 3.1 for an illustration of the supersafe bogu.

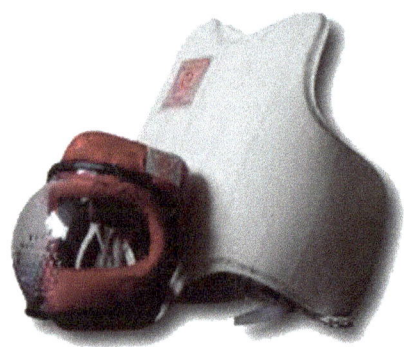

Figure 3.1: Supersafe Bogu armor, commonly used in contact fighting.

One of the main benefits of training with Bogu is that one gets to practice all the techniques on a live moving target, which forces the development of precision and an ability to anticipate small changes in distance and direction. At the same time, the Bogu has a relatively hard surface and by training techniques with it, the bones and joints of the hands can be strengthened and can become denser creating a harder, stronger fist. The muscles and tendons of the hands can also become accustomed to tightening upon impact in order to absorb the stress on the bones and joints without injury to the hand.

The Makiwara, a standing flat board used for training striking techniques has also been used by generations of karateka for the same purpose. However, it does not provide the realistic movement and targeting that is possible for a person wearing Bogu. Of course, heavy bags, hand pads, tai pads, and other commonly used striking equipment are good but they do have certain limitations in terms of replicating the movement, distancing, and targeting of a real fighting opponent. They are also not intended for training bare handed and are more suited to fight training that requires the use of boxing gloves. Training with Bogu is also beneficial as both partners can wear Bogu and practice back and forth techniques, combinations as well as offensive and defensive techniques. In short, training techniques and concepts using Bogu greatly helps to bridge the gap between training and actual fighting. It increases power and precision timing and builds fluidity in all movements and combinations while building and strengthening the body's natural weapons.

3.3 PUNCHING TECHNIQUES

There are indeed many different punching techniques used in contact fighting and self-defense such as straight punches, hook punches, uppercuts etc. Boxers and kick-boxers have developed a variety of techniques that utilize different directions and angles of attack. However, for the purpose of this book, I will provide a detailed discussion on the straight punches as well as how to build and develop them. Hook punches and uppercuts are the specialty of boxers and will not be discussed in this book. However, comparable Karate striking techniques such as chopping, ridge hand, back fist, and elbow will be discussed later in this chapter.

3.3.1 STRAIGHT PUNCHING TECHNIQUES

When executing straight punching techniques, there are some common principles that should be understood regardless of whether one is using their lead hand or back hand. Firstly, the hand's position upon contact is a key aspect. Typically, most people rotate their fist into a horizontal position upon impact, focusing the contact onto the major knuckles of their index and middle fingers. It is my opinion that this rotation of the fist when punching was mainly developed for the purpose of boxing where the fighter is wearing boxing gloves. In this way, the rotation of the fist accentuates the extra weight of the glove adding more power to the punch. At the same time, a fighter often uses a wrap to stabilize the wrist and hand and therefore, may not be as concerned with its stability. When the fist is in the horizontal position and the wrist is pointing down, the bones of the forearm cross and the wrist is not in its strongest position. At the same time, the metacarpal bones of the hands are not fully supported and can be subject to injury upon impact. It is therefore recommended that when developing barehanded punching techniques that a fighter use more of a vertical fist position upon impact, also locking the wrist with the knuckles of the index and middle fingers pointing slightly downward, as shown in Figure 3.2. This is also the same hand position used by marksmen when firing a handgun which exerts a powerful force upon firing, where the hand and wrist is well supported. By using this hand position when making contact, the hand, wrist, elbow, shoulder, and body all stay in line with the target allowing support for riving the body weight through the target. When the fist is rotated horizontally, the elbow automatically flares outward and off the target line, creating a gap between the fist and the body, therefore compromising one's ability to drive the body weight through the target.

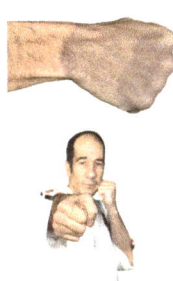

Figure 3.2: Recommended fist position for developing barehanded punching techniques. A fighter must use more of a vertical fist position upon impact, also locking the wrist with the knuckles of the index and middle fingers pointing slightly downward.

Another important concept affecting punching techniques is the positioning of the body weight depending on which hand one is using to punch with. In short, when punching, one foot is used for driving the body weight and the other foot is used for steering the body weight. To determine which foot to use for driving and which foot to use for steering, one must pay careful attention to the body's natural movement. For instance, during the movement of walking, one naturally swings their arms. In particular, as one steps forward with their left foot, one naturally swings their right arm forward and their left arm backwards. If a person tries to force themselves to walk in such a manner where one swings their left arm forward while stepping forward with the left foot, it will immediately feel unnatural and awkward. From this observation, it is clear that as one places their body weight onto the left foot, their right arm will naturally move forward, and the same is true for the other side. In this way, when punching with the lead hand, the body weight is focused from the back foot and when punching with the back hand, the body weight is focused from the front foot, while the knees are pointed towards the target. The steering foot determines the direction that the body weight is traveling. Therefore, the steering foot should always have the toes pointing in the direction of the target such that the body weight is directed at the target.

For straight punching techniques, rotation of the hips and shoulders and how they can maximize extension and power are also key aspects for consideration. The ability to rotate the body is greatly affected by the posture of the upper body. In this way, the upper body should be kept vertical to the ground in order to allow it to rotate in the direction of the target. If the upper body becomes tilted when executing a straight punch, it will result in a redirection of the body weight and thus, a loss in power and balance. In addition, the hips and shoulders should be fully extended so that at the end of the punch, one's fist and both shoulders form a straight line to the target. When executing this hip and shoulder turn, it is important to use both sides of the body to generate the momentum. In other words, while one shoulder is being rotated towards the target the other must be pulled back to generate more momentum. This is sometimes referred to as "push pull" where one side of the body is pushing (punching side) and the other side is pulling at the same time, thereby creating a centripetal force. See Figures 3.3 and 3.4 (below) for an illustration of the hip and shoulders rotation.

HIP AND SHOULDERS ROTATION

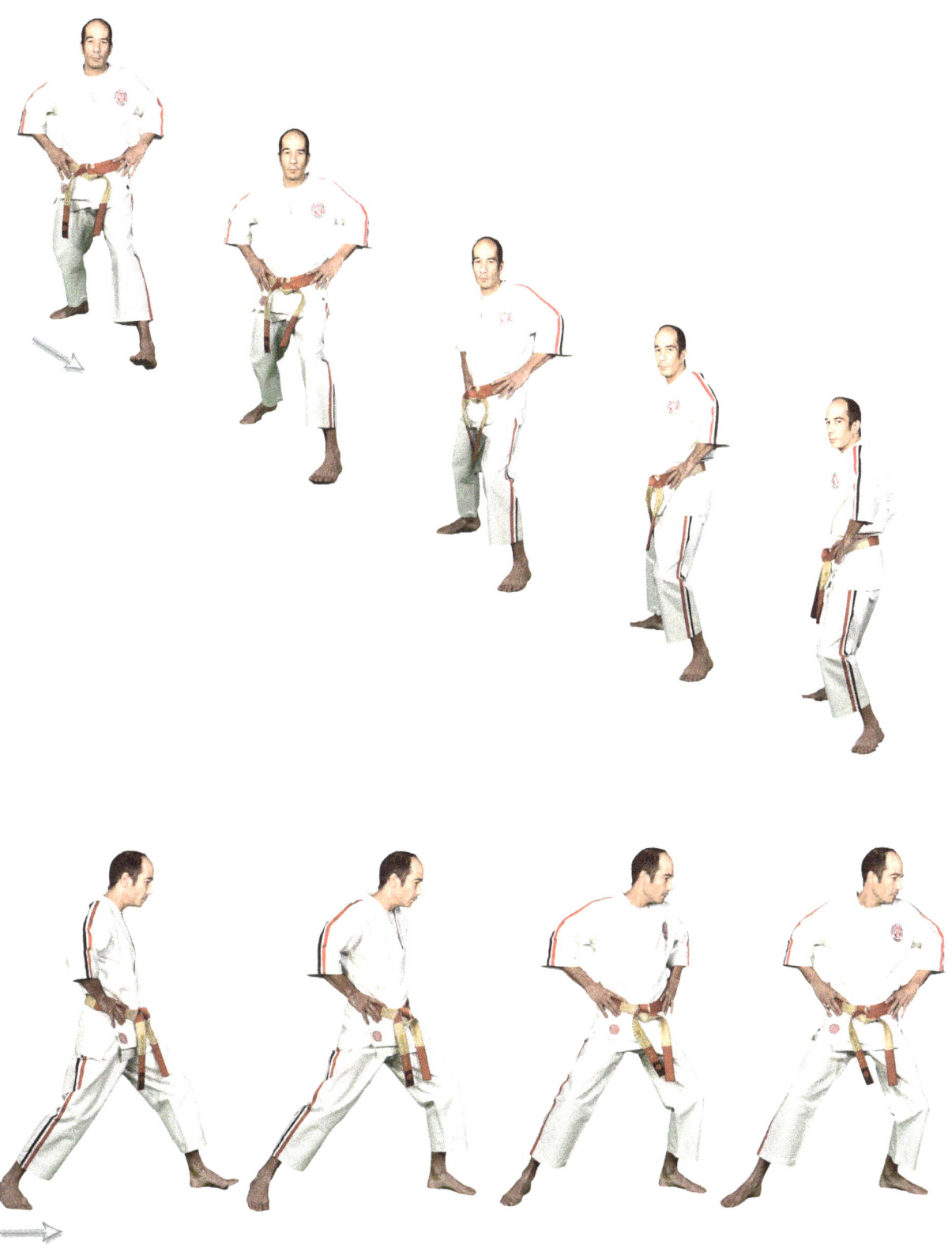

Figure 3.3: Illustration of the hip and shoulders rotation.

HIP AND SHOULDERS ROTATION

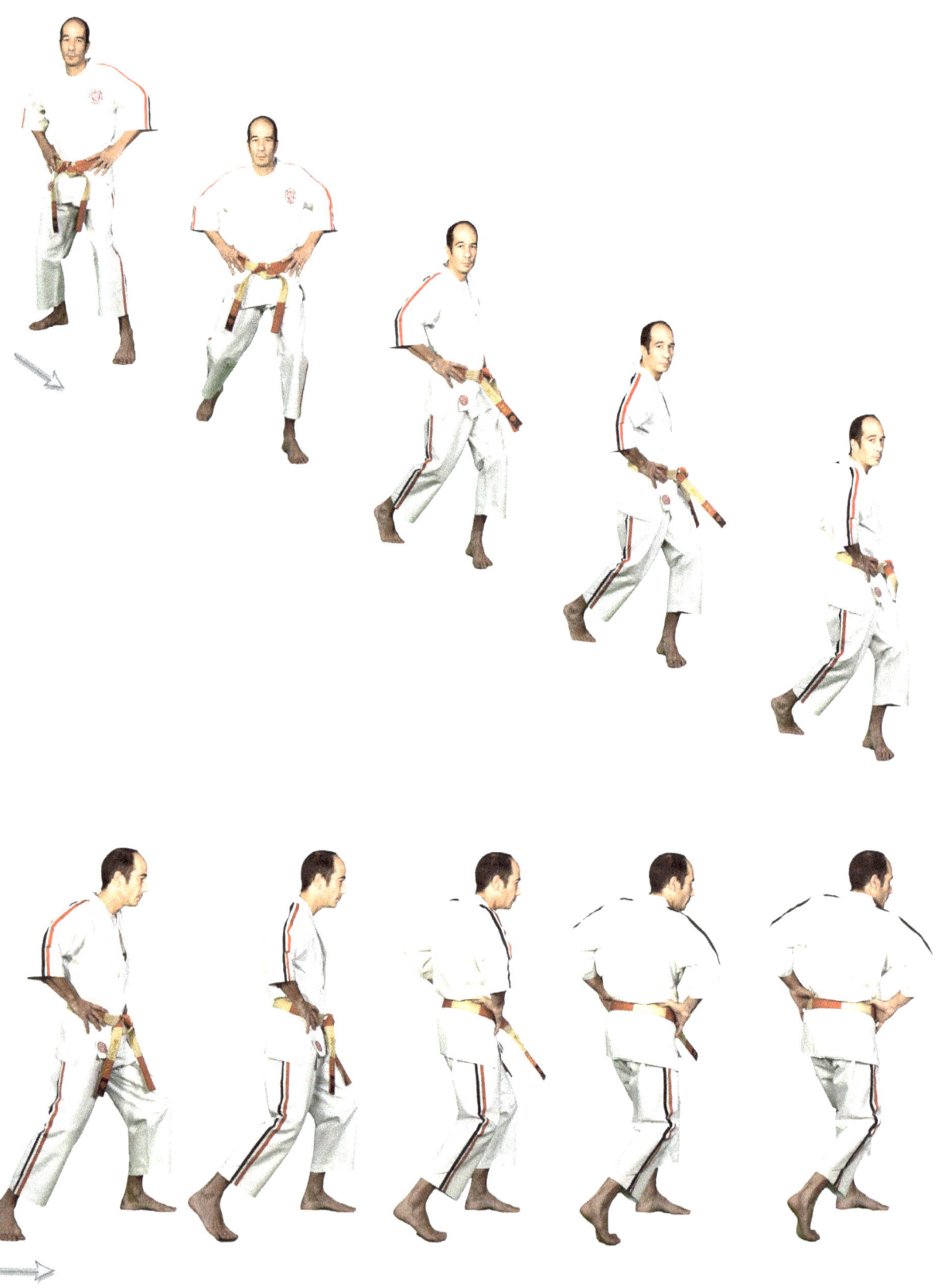

Figure 3.4: Illustration of the hip and shoulders rotation.

3.3.2 SHOMEN TSUKI (THE FRONT PUNCH - PUNCHING FROM A NATURAL STANCE)

As discussed previously in Chapter 2 on stances, the natural stance is the natural way to stand with the feet shoulder width apart. It is important to build one's punching ability from this position mainly because it forces one to deliver the power from the hips and from a much closer range than when punching from a fighting stance. Practicing this punch will teach one's body to lead the punch allowing one to deliver a lot of power from a close range.

The ability to punch effectively from this position is also very important for street self-defense as most confrontations happen from this position. While positioned in a natural stance facing front to the target, one must start the punch by pivoting on the ball of the left foot, turning the heel out and away from the body. This starts the turning of the hips clockwise towards the target, which is then followed by the extending of the fist into the target. As mentioned earlier, it is important to keep the punching arm and fist relaxed during this motion and tighten them upon contact to maximize acceleration of the fist. One can think of this entire technique like a whip or wave that starts with the turning of the foot, moves up the leg into the hips, through the shoulders, out the arm, into the fist, and into the target. After contact is made and extension is achieved, the fist must be immediately relaxed and pulled back to its starting position by retracting the hips and shoulders back to their starting position. For right punch, one must perform all the same actions in an opposite manner to that descried above. See Figures 3.5 and 3.6 (below) and the accompanying video for an illustration of the front punch.

SHOMEN TSUKI: FRONT VIEW

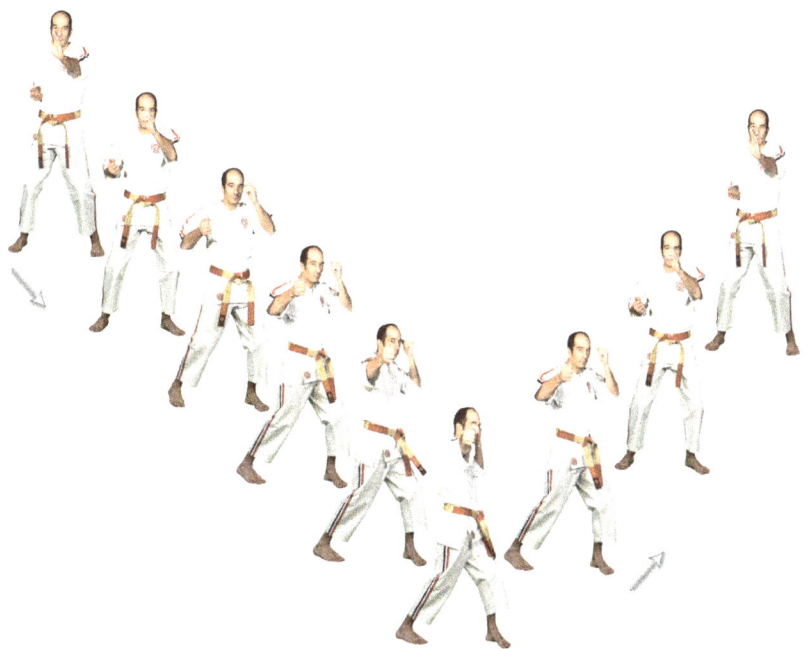

Figure 3.6: Illustrations of the Shomen Tsuki (The Front Punch - Punching from a Natural Stance), from the front view.

SHOMEN TSUKI: SIDE VIEW

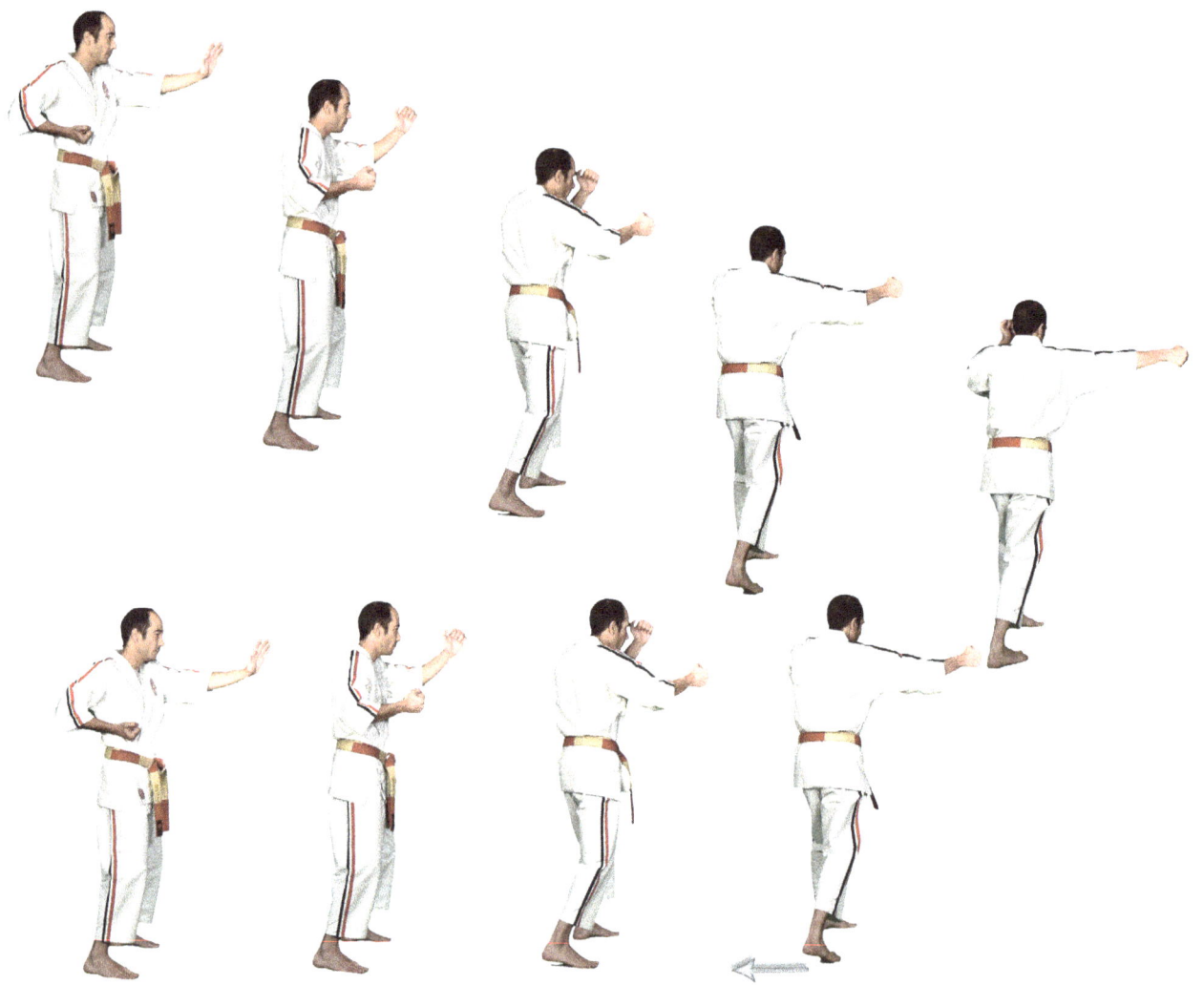

Figure 3.7: Illustrations of the Shomen Tsuki (The Front Punch - Punching from a Natural Stance), from the side view.

3.3.3 CHOKU TSUKI (STRAIGHT PUNCH, JAB, OR PUNCHING WITH THE LEAD HAND).

Almost all fighting styles have a version of the straight punch technique. For example, it is popularly used in boxing and kick boxing mainly as a lead in or distancing technique or to keep an opponent at distance however, when executed with the weight of the body, this technique can be thrown with maximum power for a much stronger effect.

From a left fighting stance centered to the target, one must push off the right foot, stepping forward with the left foot and placing it in line with the left side of the opponent's body, keeping one's centerline centered with the target. One must start with the rotation of the hips and shoulders clockwise towards the target. In the same way as the above-described front punch, the fist must then extended into the target, tightening on contact and forming a straight line from the fist to the back shoulder. For maximum power to be achieved, contact should be timed so that it occurs just before one's body weight settles on the left foot. It is also important to pay close attention to one's alignment when executing punching techniques, making sure to keep the target centered in one's stance so that the punch is also centered. As mentioned above, once contact is made and extension is achieved, the fist must be immediately relaxed and pulled back to its starting position by retracting the hips and shoulders back to their starting position. From a right fighting stance, one must perform all actions in the opposite manner to those described above. See Figures 3.8 and 3.9 (below) and the accompanying video for an illustration of Choku Tsuki.

CHOKU TSUKI (STRAIGHT PUNCH, JAB, OR PUNCHING WITH THE LEAD HAND): FRONT VIEW

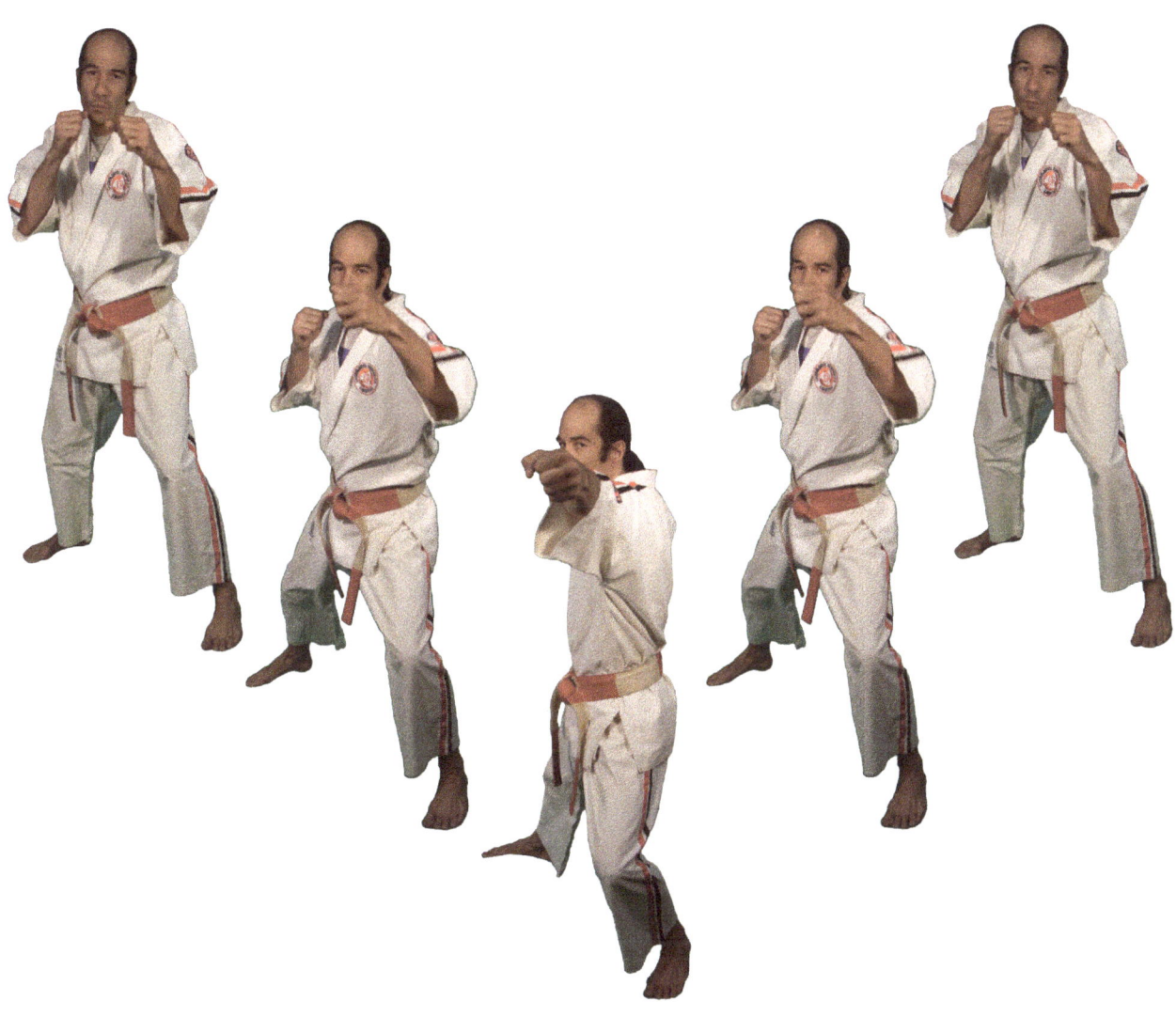

Figure 3.8: Illustrations of the Choku Tsuki, from the front view.

CHOKU TSUKI (STRAIGHT PUNCH, JAB, OR PUNCHING WITH THE LEAD HAND): SIDE VIEW

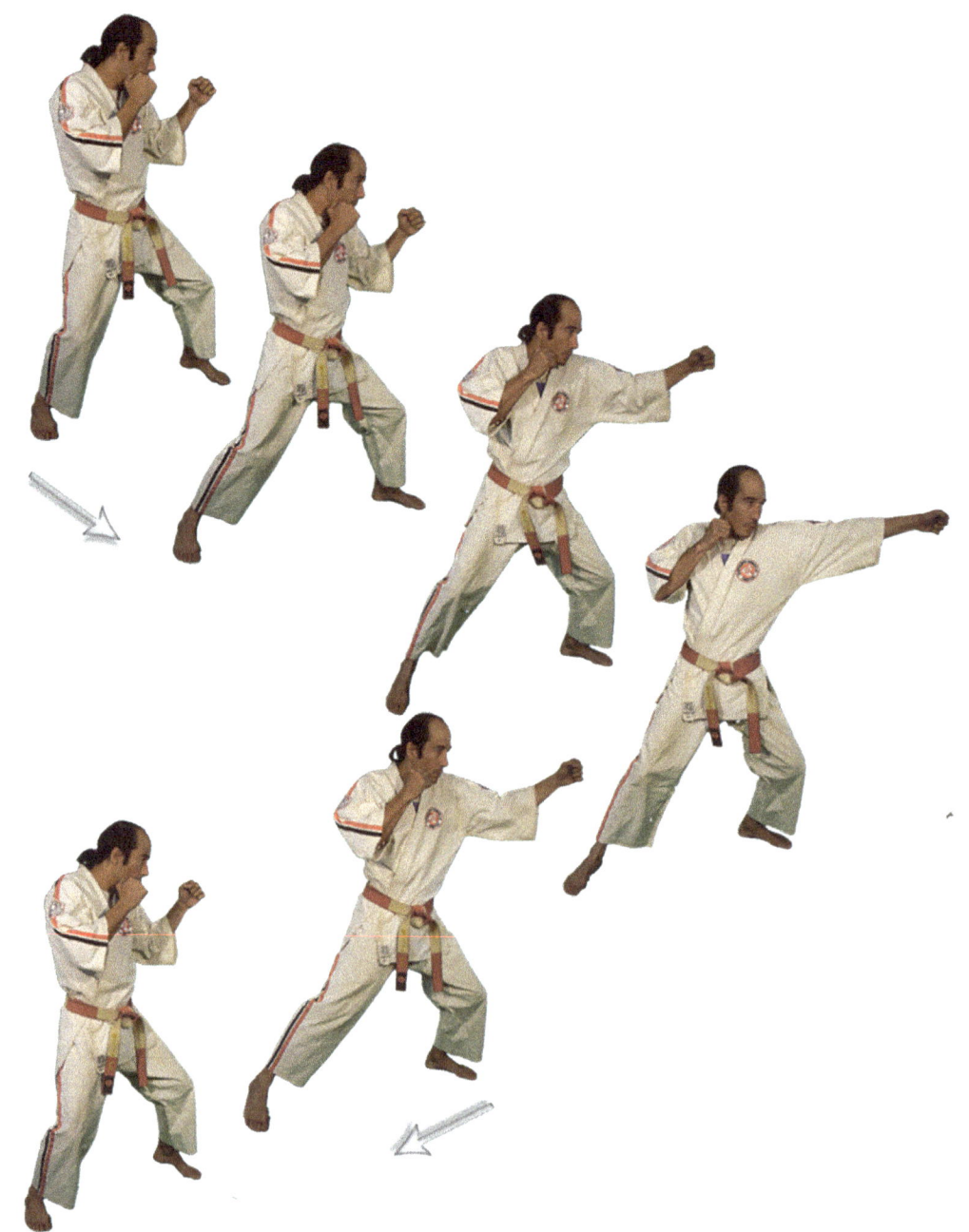

Figure 3.9: Illustrations of the Choku Tsuki, from the side view.

3.3.4 HINERI TSUKI (TWIST PUNCH, REVERSE PUNCH, CROSS OR PUNCHING WITH THE BACK HAND)

Another technique that is universal to all styles of fighting is known as Hineri Tsuki. This punch affords one with the opportunity to generate the most amount of force as it allows for the generation of a higher speed and momentum. From a left fighting stance centered to the target, one should push off with the right foot stepping forward and the left foot supporting the body weight. In addition, one must immediately start the rotation of the hips and shoulders in a counter clockwise direction towards the target. The fist must then be extended into the target, tightening on contact and forming a straight line from the right fist to the left shoulder. Power can be maximized by properly timing the contact at the moment one's body weight is settled onto the left foot. As with all punching techniques, one must also pay close attention to posture and alignment of their body. Once contact is made and extension is achieved, the fist must be immediately relaxed and pulled back to its starting position by retracting the hips and shoulders back to their starting position. From a right fighting stance, one must perform all actions in an opposite manner to those described above. See Figure 3.10 and 3.11 and the accompanying video for an illustration of Hineri Tsuki.

HINERI TSUKI: FRONT VIEW

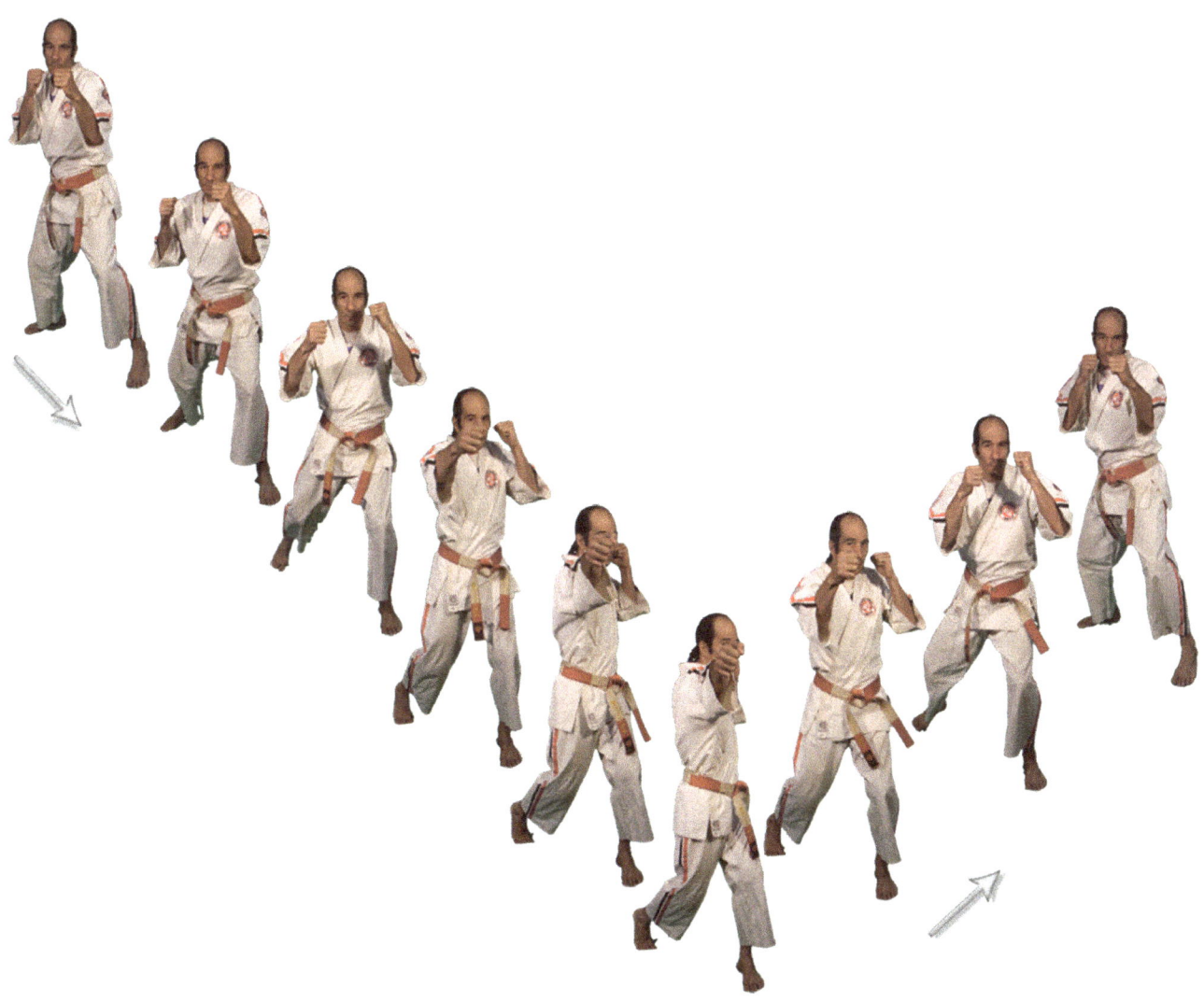

Figure 3.10: Illustrations of the Hineri Tsuki, from the front view.

HINERI TSUKI: SIDE VIEW

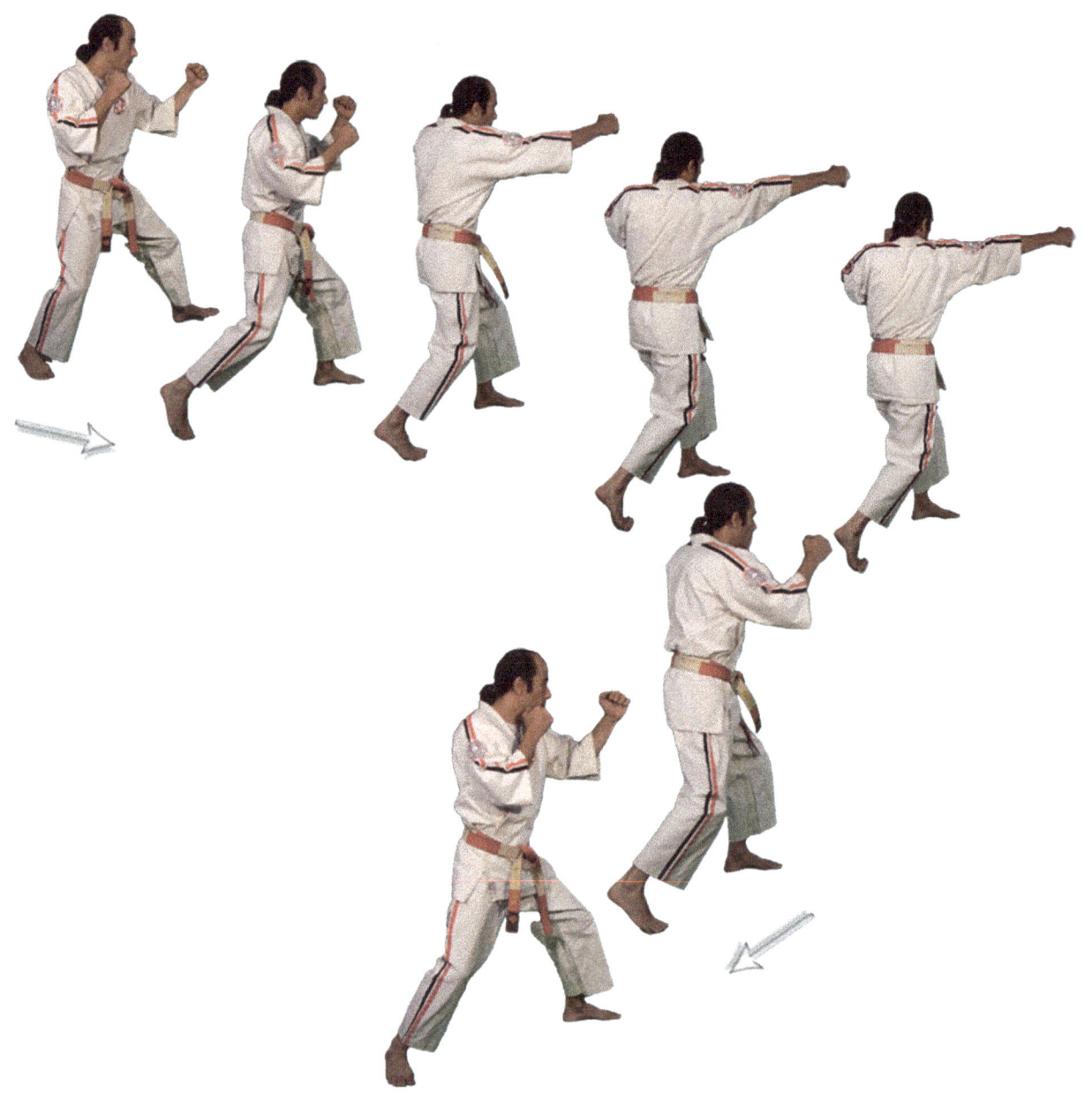

Figure 3.11: Illustrations of the Hineri Tsuki, from the side view.

3.4 KICKING TECHNIQUES

Kicking techniques are a very important aspect of martial arts training, especially for realistic contact fighting. Kicking techniques can increase a fighter's striking range and deliver more power than hand techniques however, they are not without additional risks. When executing a kick, one must balance their body weight on one foot thus, making it easier to have their balance affected. At the same time, being on one foot limits mobility and can make it difficult to defend a counterattack. For this reason, it is very important to develop kicking techniques that maximize power but also balance the body weight in the most efficient way so as to create good balance throughout the delivery of the kick.

For the most part, kicking techniques fall into one of three categories, namely _straight/front kicks, round kicks, and side kicks_. As with punching techniques, to maximize the power of kicking techniques, one must drive the techniques with the weight of the whole body. This is done by either thrusting, turning, or extending the hips and torso depending on the technique being executed. The arms can also be used in a swinging motion to add momentum to the hip and shoulder movements thus, truly using the entire body to generate the force of the technique. It is also crucial to understand that the movement of the hips and shoulders are affected by the position of the supporting foot in any kicking technique. It is therefore vital for a trainee to develop a proper understanding of the different foot positions and body movements as they relate to each type of kicking technique. In addition, for all kicking techniques, the posture of the spine will directly affect one's ability to extend their hips and drive their body weight. A straight back or spine will allow the hips and shoulders to align and therefore drive the weight of the body with the technique. Alternatively, curving or bending of the spine will impede the movement of the hips and shoulders, mainly because the hips and shoulders will no longer be on the same line and therefore cannot move as a unit to drive the body.

3.4.1 STRAIGHT KICKS

Straight kicks, also known as front kicks or push kicks are kicks delivered in a straight line to the target. They can be delivered with the front or back foot while contact can be made with the ball or heel of the foot. For this kick, the power of the technique is driven by thrusting the hips in a forward direction towards the target. To effectively accomplish this, the shoulders must be pulled backwards to counter balance the weight of the hips. In this way, the torso acts like a balancing scale that generates power and creates balance at the same time. In addition to the involvement of the hips and shoulders, the arm on the kicking side of the body must be swung out to the side of the body assisting the hips to generate momentum as it is thrusted forward towards the target. At the same time, the opposite hand must be pulled in front of the face and body, covering the centerline and protecting the vitals.

As mentioned earlier in this chapter, the thrusting of the hips is affected by the position of the supporting foot, especially the direction of the toes. For the hips to be thrusted forward, the toes of the supporting foot must be turned outward facing away from the target at an approximately 45 degrees angle. In this position, the hip socket remains open and allows the hips to thrust forward while maintaining balance on the supporting foot. An easy way to understand the effects of foot position is to place one foot on a wall at about the hip's height. Then, attempt to push the wall with the foot, either with the toes of the supporting foot facing the wall or with the toes turned away from the wall at a 45 degrees angle. Here, one will notice a considerable difference when trying to push with the toes facing the wall, whereby one's balance will be compromised forcing one up onto the ball of the foot, losing balance, and falling backwards.

It is very important for power and stability to keep the heel of the supporting foot on the ground when kicking to allow one to drive the body weight with the power of the legs and maintain balance through contact. It is also very important to time the thrusting forward of the hips at the same time as the extension of the kick. Extending the hips forward prior to extending the kick will result in the body weight not being exerted into the kick, resulting in a loss of power and ending up with a pushing kick rather than a striking penetrating kick. A similar result is also achieved if the knee is lifted higher than the target prior to extending the kick, whereby the hips are no longer in a position to drive into the target and the kick becomes a push rather that a strike.

A. Shomen Mae Geri (Straight kick from the Natural Stance)

As discussed previously in Chapter 2 on stances, the natural stance is the natural way to stand with the feet positioned at shoulders width apart. It is important to build one's kicking ability from this position mainly because it forces one to deliver the power from the hips and legs without the assistance of momentum generated from stepping or wind-up movements and from a much closer range than when kicking from a fighting stance. Practicing this kick will train one's body to lead the kick allowing one to deliver a lot of power from a close range. The ability to kick effectively from this position is also very important for self- defense strategies in everyday life because most confrontations happen from this position.

From a natural stance facing front to the target, a fighter must start the kick by bringing the left foot close to the right foot and by turning the right foot outward at the same time so that the toes are pointing at approximately 45 degrees away from the target, while simultaneously bending the knees to lower one's center of gravity. Next, a fighter must begin to lift the heel of their left foot and then raise the knee to the height of the target. The hips must then be thrusted forward and the kick must be extended towards the target, making contact with either the heel or the ball of the foot, driving through the target by pushing the hips. It is important to note that when the hips are thrust forward, the shoulders must move backwards to counterbalance the thrusting motion of the hips. The left hand must also be extended out to the side and back at the same time, while the right hand must be used to cover the body's centerline. This will help in thrusting the hips forward, generating momentum, and creating stability and balance during the execution of the kick, allowing one to drive their body weight into the target without losing balance.

All motions in this kick must be practiced to become one fluid motion in order to maximize speed and body extension and to synchronize the timing of the thrusting of the hips with the extending of the kick. After the kick reaches full extension, a fighter must quickly retract their foot and hip, bring their shoulders back to the starting position and placing the foot back on the ground in its starting position. A fighter must perform all the above-mentioned movements in reverse for kicking with the right foot. See Figure 3.12 and the accompanying video for an illustration of the Shomen Mae Geri move and its components.

SHOMEN MAE GERI (STRAIGHT KICK FROM NATURAL STANCE)
SIDE VIEW

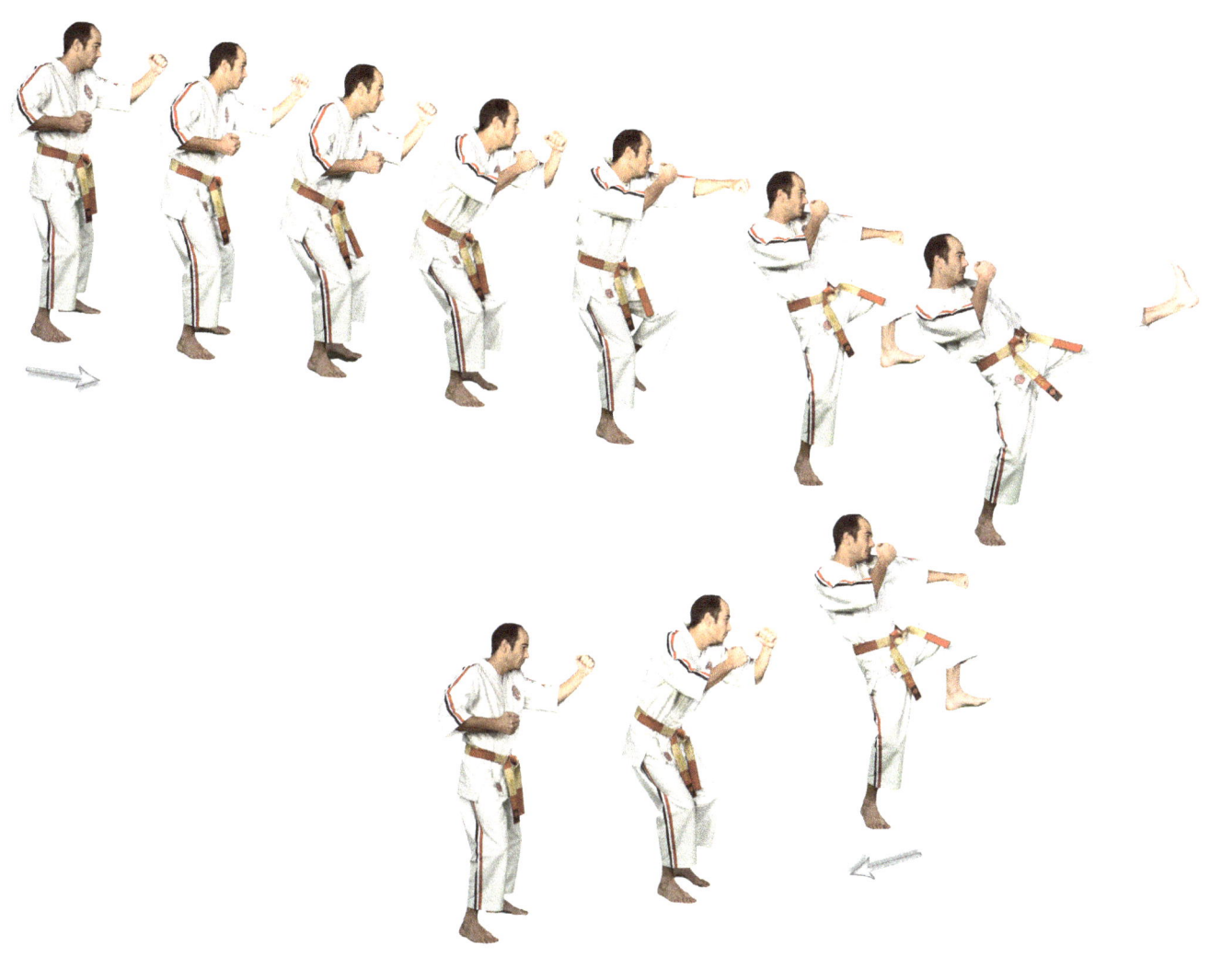

FRONT VIEW

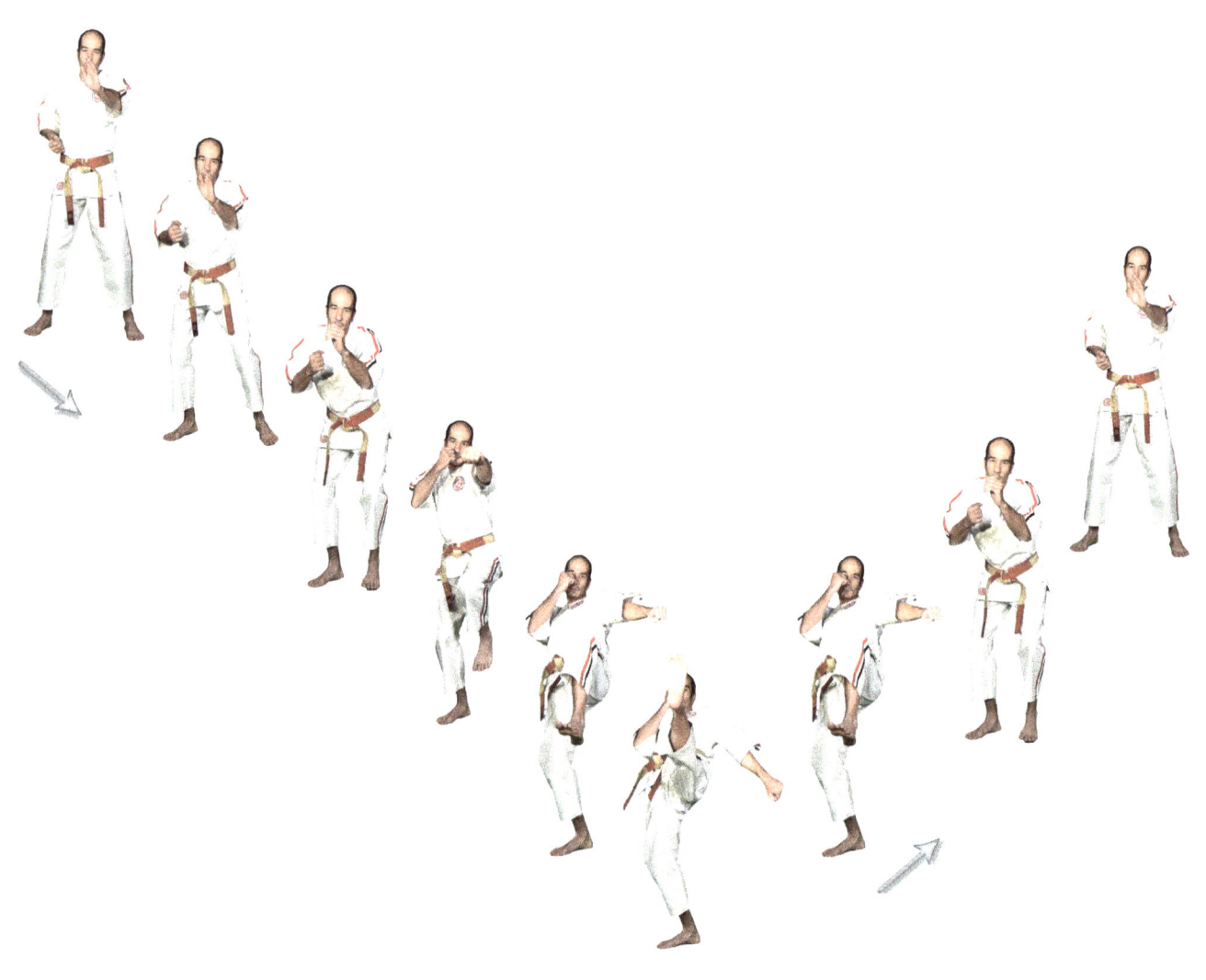

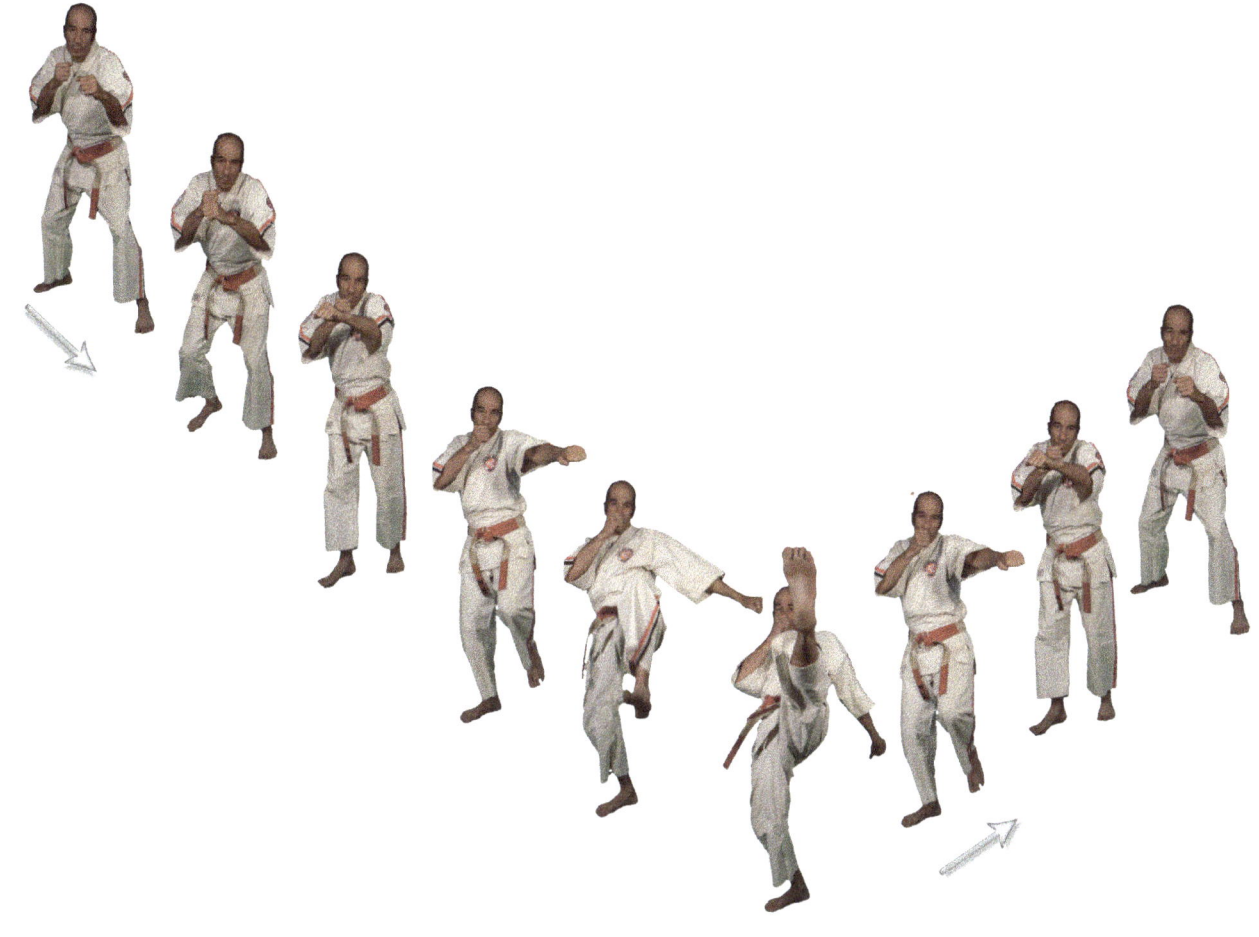

Figure 3.12: Illustrations of the Shomen Mae Geri, from the side and front views.

B. Oi Mae Geri (Lunge Front Kick, Straight Kick with the Front Foot)

From a left fighting stance centered to the target, one must bring the right foot forward as far as necessary to be at a kicking distance from the target. The size of this step will vary depending on how far one is standing from the target, with their toes facing away from the target at approximately 45 degrees and knees slightly bent to lower the center of gravity. Next, a fighter must begin lifting the left foot's heel (i.e. the kicking foot's), followed by the left knee to approximately the same height as the target. The hips must then be thrusted forward and the kick must be extended towards the target, thereby making contact with either the heel or the ball of the foot and driving through the target by pushing the hips.

As with the Showmen Mae Geri move, the shoulders must move back with the thrusting of the hips and the left arm must be swung to the side and back to help with maintaining balance and generating momentum, while the right hand must be brought forward to cover and protect the centerline of the body. After the kick reaches full extension, a fighter must quickly retract their foot and hips, bring the shoulders back to their starting position and placing it back on the ground close to the right foot and immediately stepping back with the right foot returning to the original fighting stance. One must perform all movements in reverse from a right fighting stance for a right lunge front kick. See Figures 3.13 and 3.14 (below) and video for illustration of Oi Mae Geri.

OI MAE GERI: FRONT VIEW

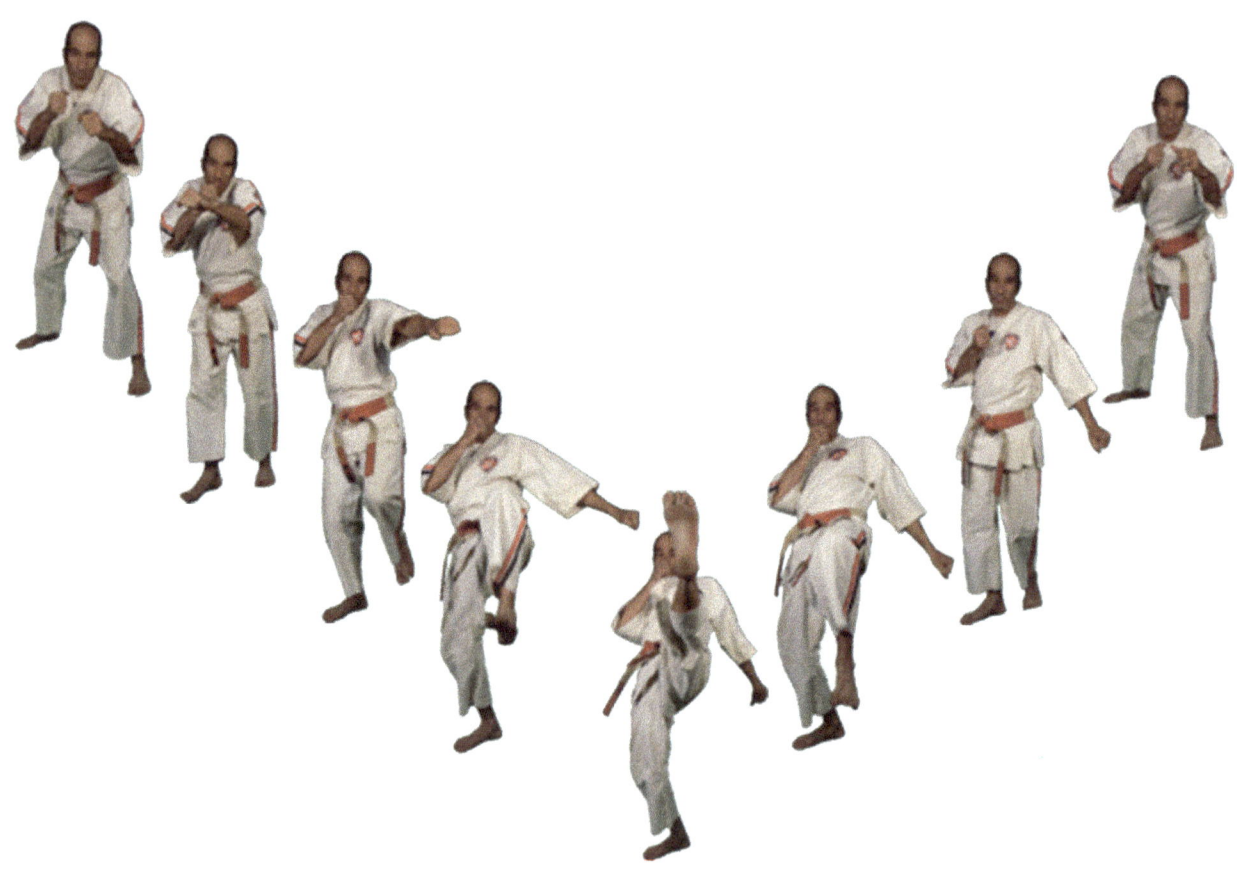

Figure 3.13: Illustrations of the Oi Mae Geri, from the front view.

OI MAE GERI: SIDE VIEW

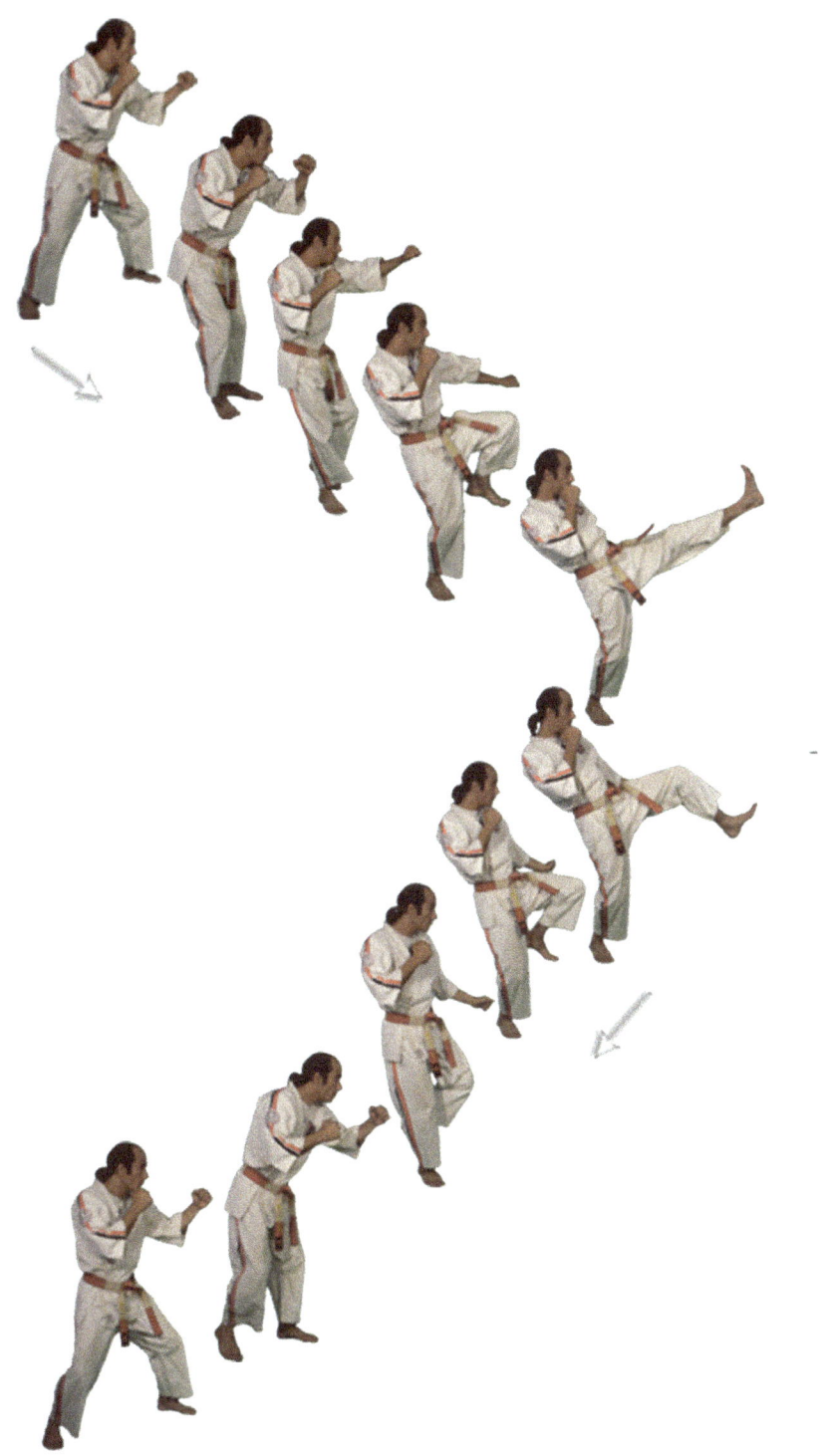

Figure 3.14: Illustrations of the Oi Mae Geri, from the side view.

C. Hineri Mae Geri (twist front kick, straight kick with the back foot)

From a left fighting stance centered to the target, one must push off the right foot stepping forward with the left foot placing it at the necessary distance from the target with the toes pointing 45 degrees away from the target and knees slightly bent to lower the center of gravity. Next, one must first begin lifting the right foot's heel (i.e. the kicking foot's), followed by raising the knee to the height of the target. The hips must then be thrusted forward and the kick must be extended towards the target, making contact with either the heel or the ball of the foot and driving through the target by pushing the hips.

As with the other straight kicks, the shoulders must move back with the thrusting of the hips and the right arm on the kicking side must be swung to the side and back to help with balance and momentum. The left hand (i.e. on the supporting foot's side) must be brought forward to cover and protect the centerline of the body. After the kick reaches full extension, one must quickly retract the foot and hips, bringing the shoulders back to their starting position and placing the foot either back at its starting point or forward into a right fighting stance if one wishes to continue offensively. One must perform all movements in reverse from a right fighting stance for a left twist front kick. See Figures 3.15 and 3.16 (below) and video for illustration of Hineri Mae Geri.

HINERI MAE GERI: FRONT VIEW

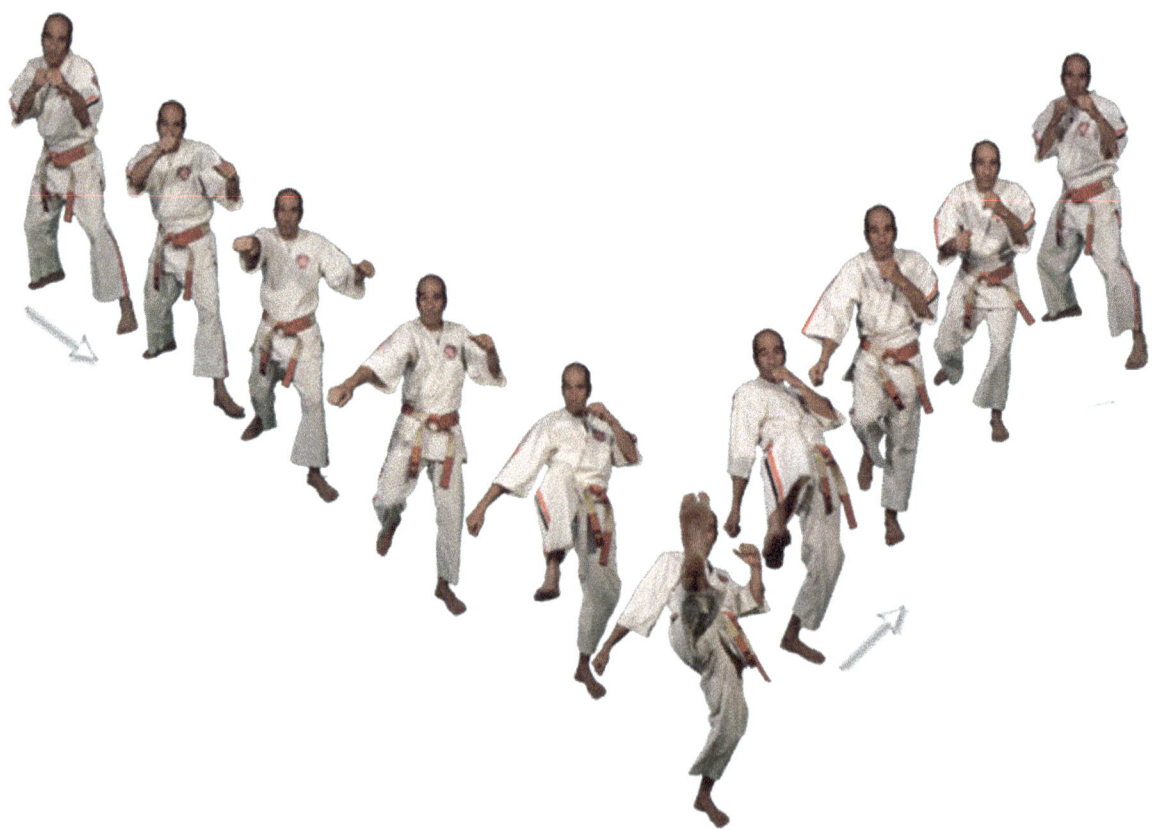

Figure 3.15: Illustrations of the Hineri Mae Geri, from the front view.

HINERI MAE GERI: SIDE VIEW

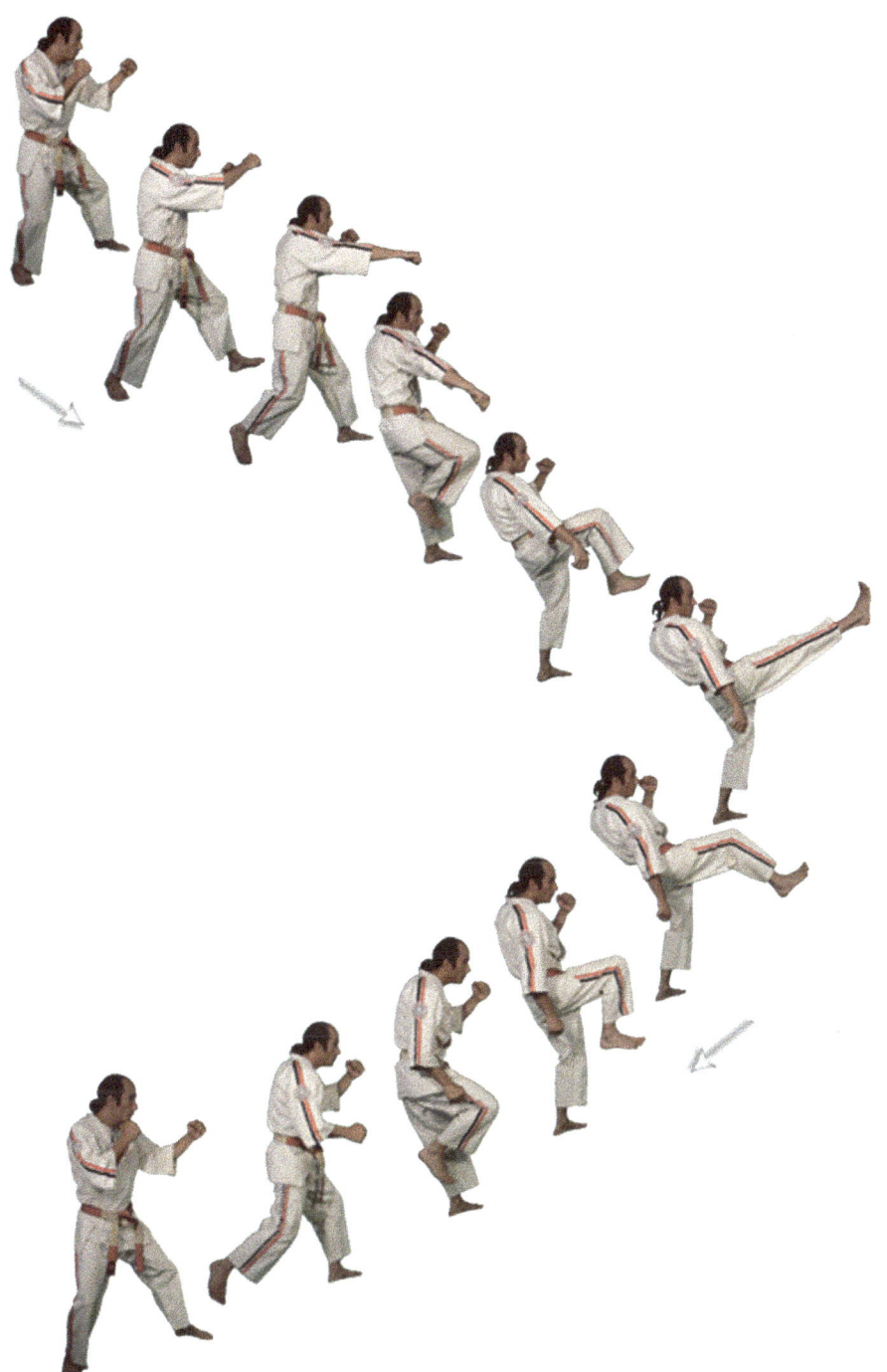

Figure 3.16: Illustrations of the Hineri Mae Geri, from the side view.

D. Yoko Geri (Side Kick)

As the name of this kick implies, the side kick must be delivered from a sideways position to the target. This is also an extremely powerful technique when delivered with the extension of the hips and body. From a left fighting stance and centered to the target, one must push off with the right foot stepping forward and place the left foot's heel on the target line, with its toes facing 90 degrees away from the target line. One must bring the right foot towards the left, placing it at the necessary distance from the target with the toes pointing in the opposite direction as that of the target placing it at the necessary distance from the target. Then, one must lift the left knee to the height of the target and keep it at a 90 degrees angle to the target. Finally, one must initiate the extension of the kick by tilting the upper body at the waist level in the opposite direction of the target and drive the heel of the foot into the target, thereby with a full extension of the left leg and upper body.

In situations where the right foot needs to pass the left foot to achieve distancing, it must be placed behind the left foot and not in front of it. When the right foot is placed in front of the left foot (i.e. kicking foot), it will force the hips to turn rather than extend sideways. After the kick has reached full extension, one must pull back the knee immediately and place the left foot back down, close to the right foot, and step back with the right foot into a left fighting stance. It is also important to note that as described above, the knee of the kicking foot must be lifted and the foot must be extended to the target. It is a common mistake made with the side kick that the foot is extended to the target without lifting the knee. If the knee is not lifted, it will inevitably turn downwards and point to the ground, forcing the kick to rise as it heads to the target. This would disconnect the hips from driving the extension of the foot resulting in a less powerful kick and usually a loss of balance. A fighter must perform all these movements in reverse manner from a right fighting stance for a right side kick. See Figures 3.17 and 3.18 below and the accompanying video for illustrations of Yoko Geri (side kick).

YOKO GERI: FRONT VIEW

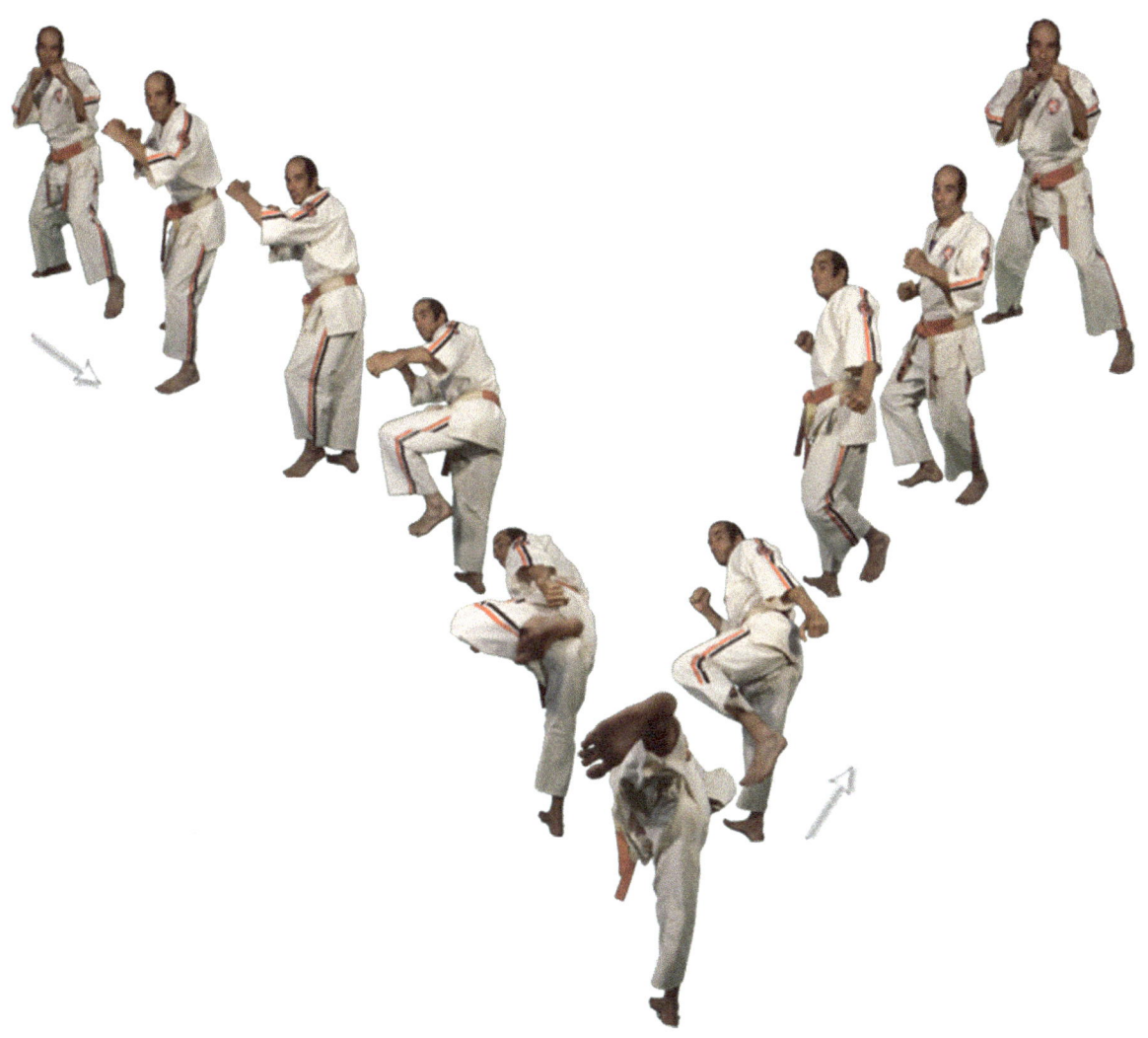

Figure 3.17: Illustrations of the Yoko Geri, from the front view.

YOKO GERI: SIDE VIEW

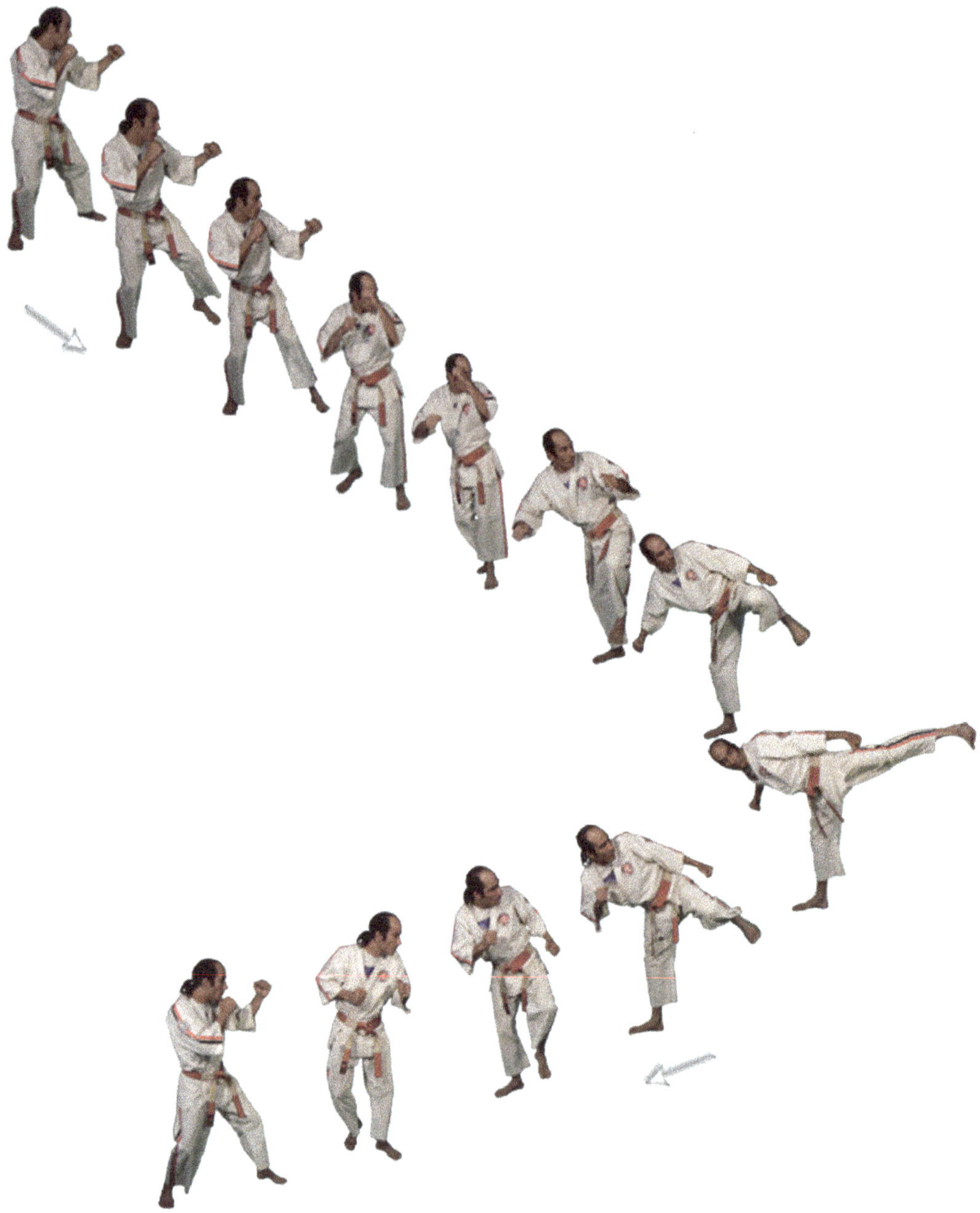

Figure 3.18: Illustrations of the Yoko Geri, from the side view.

3.4.2 ROUNDHOUSE KICKS

The most popular and widely used technique in all of martial arts is the roundhouse kick. As its name implies, it is delivered in a circular motion utilizing the hips and shoulders to drive the kick into the target. In general, contact must be made with either the instep or the lower part of the shin bone however, contact can also be made with the ball of the foot or the heel of the foot, particularly in "street type situations" where one is likely wearing shoes or boots. For the purpose of this book, I will focus on referring to the shin or instep depending on the height of the target. As a general rule, the effective distance gets longer as the target gets higher and thus requires the full length of the weapon (i.e. the kicking foot). Alternatively, the distance of the target decreases as the height of the target gets lower thus requiring shorter length of the weapon. It is recommended that when using the roundhouse kick at a low target such as the leg, a fighter must ensure that the contact is focused with the shin. Similarly, when kicking a high target such as the body, a fighter must focus contact with the lower shin and part of the upper instep. Finally, when kicking to the head target, the instep of the foot must be utilized. A variation of the roundhouse kick can also be used as a sweeping or off-balancing technique which will be outlined later in this book.

Oi Mawashi Geri (Lunge Roundhouse Kick, Roundhouse Kick with the Front Leg)

From a left fighting stance and centered to the target, one must bring the right foot forward as far as necessary to position oneself in the kicking distance from the target and place it slightly to the right of the target. In the next step, one must lift the left knee to the height of the target so that a straight line can be formed between the hip and the tip of the knee pointing slightly left of the target. This move must be performed with the knee bent and the foot pulled back towards the buttocks. Then, one must start extending the kick towards the target by pivoting on the ball of the foot and dropping the body weight on the heel. The foot should be pivoted until its heel lines up with the target so that the hips and shoulders can rotate past the target line. As soon as the foot begins to pivot, one must pull the shoulders backwards to create an angle with the upper body and the trunk, in order to counter balance the extension of the leg.

Simultaneously, one must also start rotating the hips and shoulders in a clockwise direction and release the hinge of the knee driving the kick into the target. The shoulders and hips should be rotated until they pass the target line. This will ensure that the weight of the body has been driven through the target. The timing of this kick must be practiced so that contact is made at the same time as the body weight is dropped on the heel of the pivoting foot and the left shoulder just passes through the target line. After fully extending the kick, one must quickly pull back the foot by bending the knee and simultaneously re-pivoting the supporting foot and re-placing the heel to its start point. Then one must place the kicking foot close to the supporting foot and step back with the supporting foot into a left fighting stance. One must perform all of the above-mentioned movements in a reverse manner from a right fighting stance for a right lunge roundhouse kick.

Note: To perform this technique from a close range, where stepping forward with the back foot is not possible, one can use the distancing step, switching both feet at the same time. This would aid with adjusting the distance of the supporting foot without stepping forward and ending up too close to the target. The kick must be executed as described above. In sum, the switching step places a fighter in the same position as stepping forward with the back foot but does it from a close range. See Figures 3.19 and 3.20 and the accompanying video for detailed illustrations of Oi Mawashi Geri.

OI MAWASHI GERI: SIDE VIEW

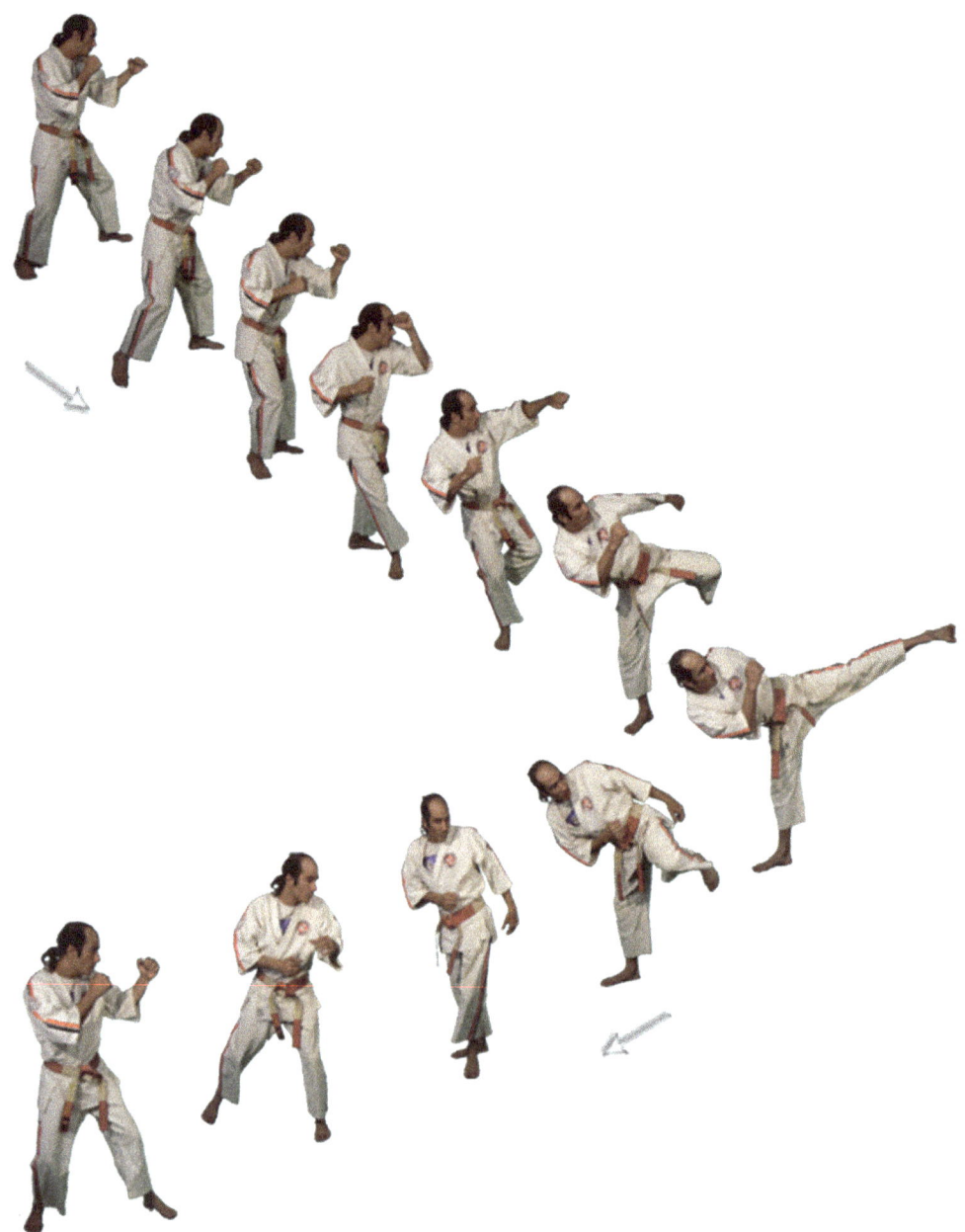

Figure 3.19: Illustrations of Oi Mawashi Geri, from the side view.

OI MAWASHI GERI: FRONT VIEW

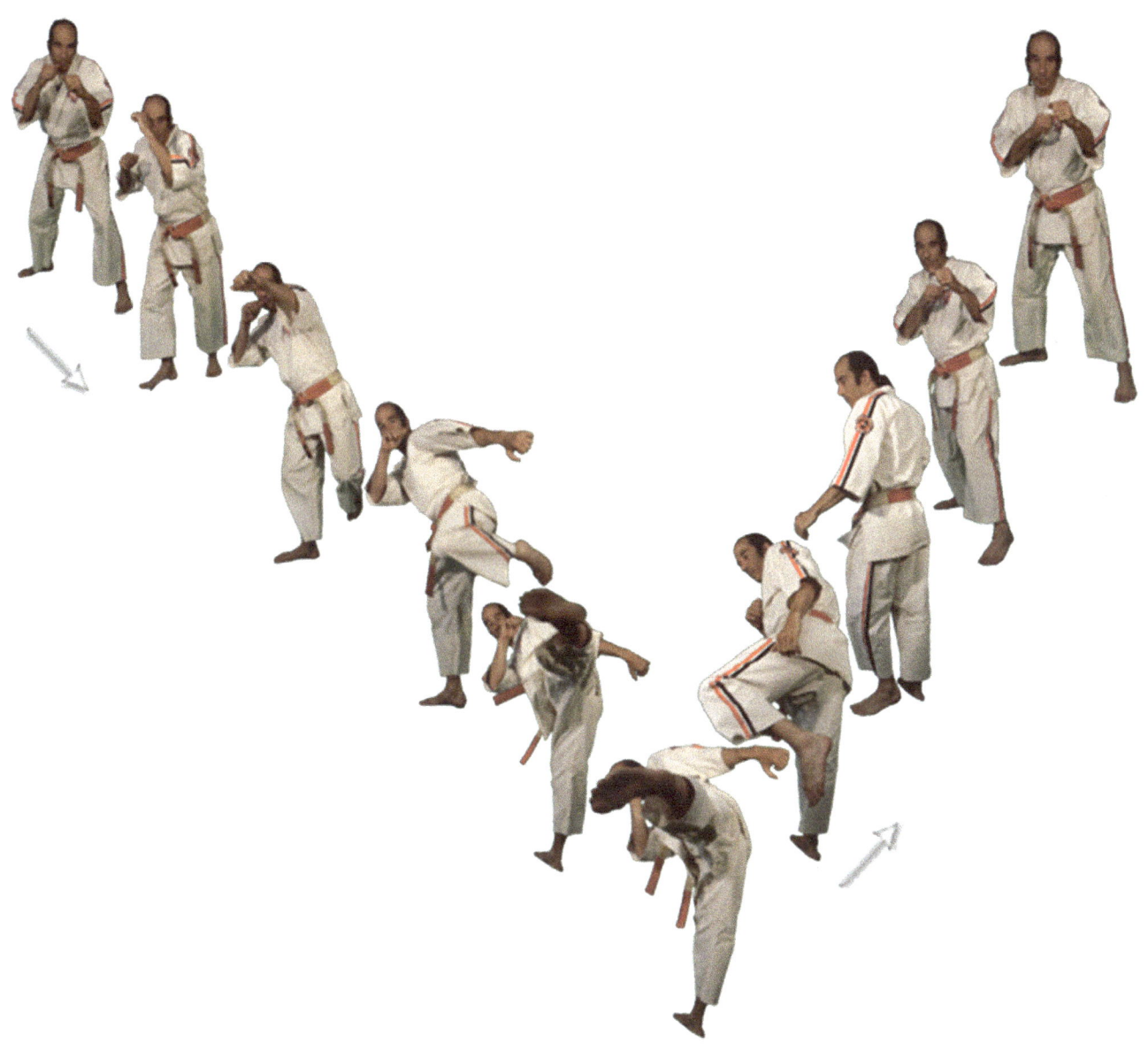

Figure 3.20: Illustrations of Oi Mawashi Geri, from the side view.

Hineri Mawashi Geri (Twist Roundhouse Kick, Swing Round House Kick, Roundhouse Kick with the Back Leg)

The roundhouse kick with the back leg is probably the most commonly used technique in all fighting competitions. It shares the same mechanics as the front leg and requires the pivoting of the supporting foot to allow the hips and shoulders to rotate through the target and maximize power.

From a left fighting stance and centered to the target, a fighter must push off the right leg stepping forward and slightly left of the target with the left foot toes pointing slightly left of the target, thereby placing it at the correct distance from the target to deliver the roundhouse kick with the right leg.

Next, one must lift the knee of the right foot (i.e. kicking foot) to the height in which a straight line is made from the hip to the tip of the knee and points to the height of the target and slightly right of the target, with the knee bent and the foot pulled back towards the buttocks. Next, one must begin with the extending of the kick by first pivoting on the ball of the supporting foot (i.e. left foot) and swinging the heel of this foot towards the target dropping the body weight on the heel and timing it with the moment of contact. The foot should be pivoted until its heel lines up with the target so that the hips and shoulders can rotate past the target line. As soon as the foot begins to pivot, one must pull the shoulders backwards to create an angle with the upper body and the trunk so as to counter balance the extension of the leg and simultaneously start rotating the hips and shoulders in a counter clockwise direction.

Lastly, one must release the hinge of the knee driving the kick into the target. The shoulders and hips should be rotated until they just pass the target line to ensure that the weight of the body has been driven through the target. The timing of this kick must be practiced so that contact is made just as the body weight is dropped on the heel of the pivoting foot and the left shoulder just passes through the target line. After fully extending the kick, one must quickly pull back the foot by bending the knee. One must also simultaneously re-pivot the supporting foot replacing the heel where it started, then placing the kicking foot back to its starting position in a left fighting stance. A fighter must perform all movements in reverse from a right fighting stance for a left twist roundhouse kick. See Figures 3.21 and 3.22 below and the accompanying video for illustration of Hineri Mawashi Geri.

HINERI MAWASHI GERI: FRONT VIEW

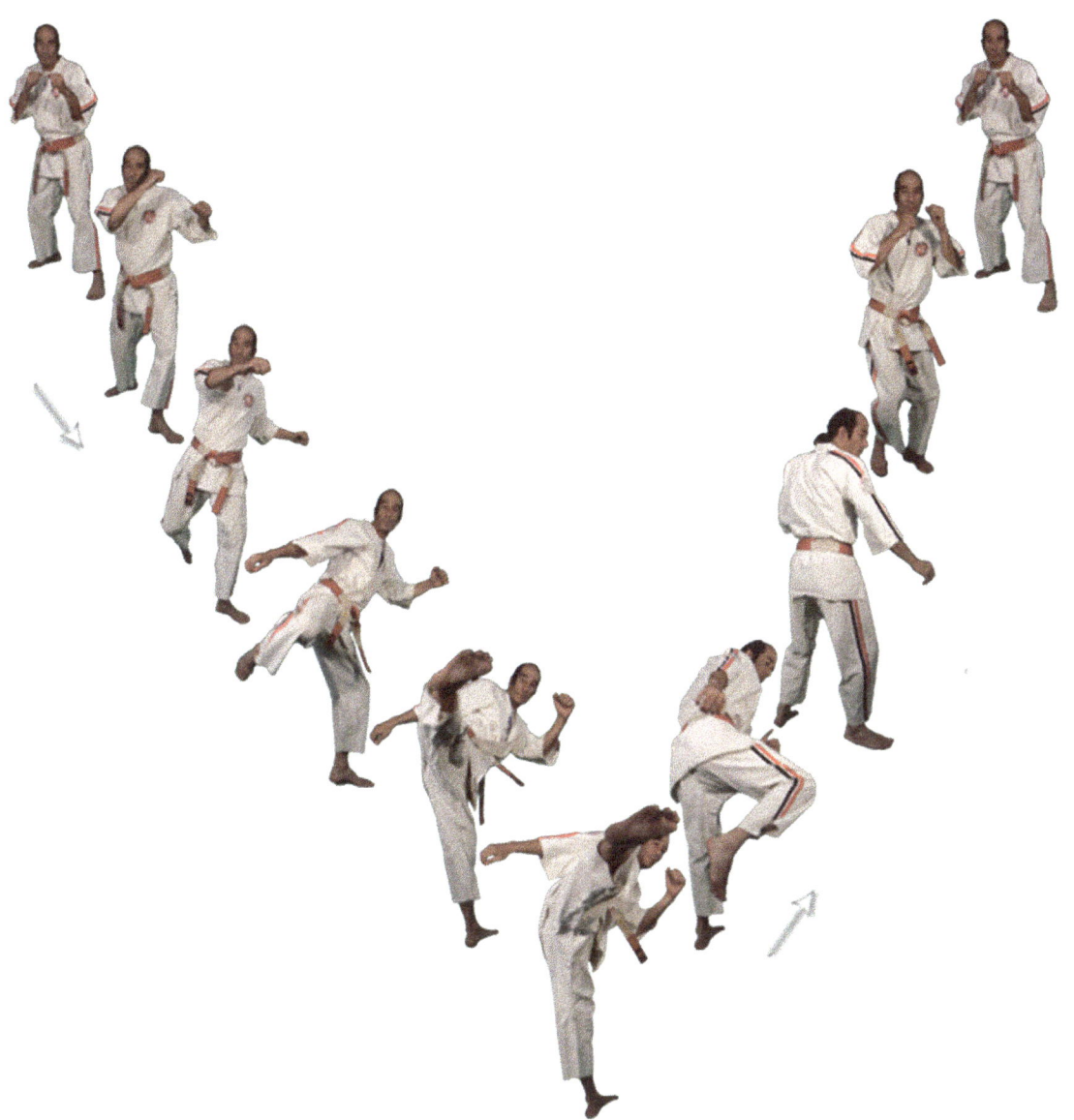

Figure 3.21: Illustrations of Hineri Mawashi Geri, from the front view.

HINERI MAWASHI GERI: SIDE VIEW

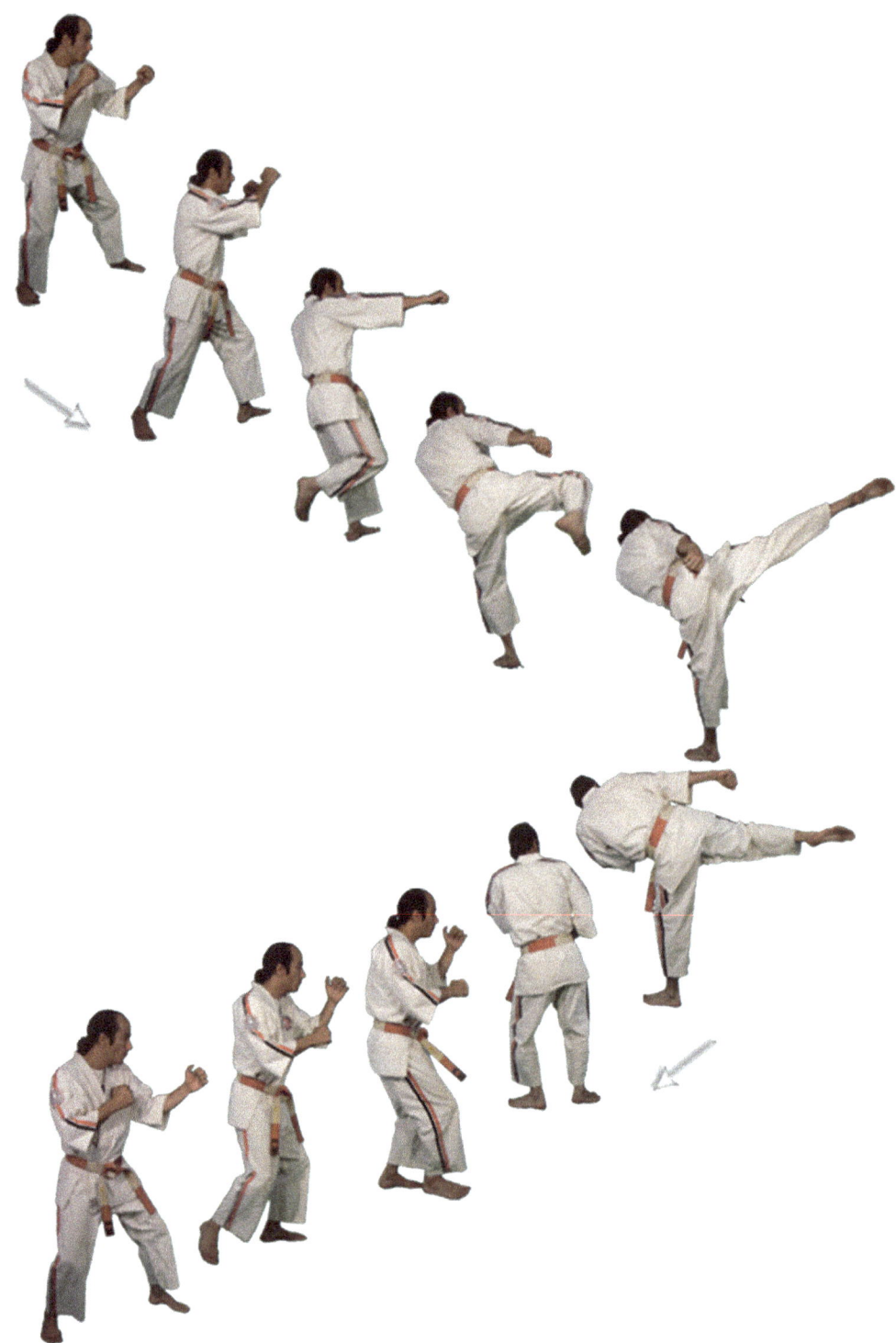

Figure 3.22: Illustrations of Hineri Mawashi Geri, from the side view.

Ushiro Mawashi Geri (Back Roundhouse Kick, Spinning Back Kick, Back Wheel Kick)

The back roundhouse kick is a very popular kicking technique in part because it is probably the most impressive looking technique and has been popularized in martial arts films. In reality, it is also a very powerful and effective technique that has been used with great success in professional fighting arenas around the world. Although there are many little variations in how this technique is performed from style to style, the basic mechanics are universal and as all other techniques, this one also requires the turning and extending of the hips and shoulders to drive the kick into the target. During this kick, contact is generally made with the bottom or back side of the heels of the foot depending on whether the target is the opponent's body or head. A fighter must mainly focus on making contact with the bottom of the heel when kicking to the opponent's body and making contact with the back of the heel when kicking to the opponent's head. For this purpose, the technique must be delivered in a more circular way when kicking to the opponent's head and delivered in a straight way when kicking to the opponent's body. The hips and shoulders must be rotated in the same way regardless of the target.

From a left fighting stance centered to the target, one must push off the right leg stepping forward with the left foot (i.e. supporting foot), placing it slightly past the target line with its toes facing 90 degrees away from the target line and at the necessary distance from the target to effectively deliver the kick. Next, one must pivot both feet clockwise and turn the hips and shoulders and head until the shoulders and hips are square to the target and one is looking over their right shoulder directly at the target. Next one must lift the knee of the right leg with the knee bent at approximately 90 degrees and continue with the clockwise turning of the hips and shoulders in order to extend the kick towards the target, thereby driving it with the turning of the hips and shoulders. Finally, one must extend their body in a straight line upon contact, driving through the target with the bottom of the heel. After full extension, one must pull the foot back by bending the knee and continue with the rotation of the hips and shoulders all the way around and step back with the right foot into a left fighting stance.

For a back roundhouse kick to the head, one must extend the kick as described however, one must begin extending the kick slightly to the left of the target and allow the turning of the hips to bring it into the target, making contact with the back of the heel just as the leg reaches full extension. Then, pull the heel through the target by bending the knee and continuing with the rotation of the hips and shoulders through the target and completely around stepping back into the original left fighting stance.

Note: It is important to allow the left foot (i.e. supporting foot) to pivot freely throughout the execution of this technique to allow for smooth turning of the hips and shoulders and to allow for the weight of the body to drive the technique through the target.

It is also important to note that as with a side kick, it is essential to lift the knee of the kicking foot before extending the kick so as to align the hips with the extension of the kick. It is a common mistake made with the back roundhouse kick and the side kick, whereby the foot is extended to the target without lifting the knee. When this is done, the knee turns downwards and points to the ground, disconnecting the hips from driving the extension of the foot resulting in a less powerful kick and usually a loss of balance. One must perform all movements in reverse from a right fighting stance for a left back roundhouse kick. See Figures 3.23 and 3.24 and the accompanying video for illustrations of Ushiro Mawashi Geri to the body and head.

USHIRO MAWASHI GERI: FRONT VIEW

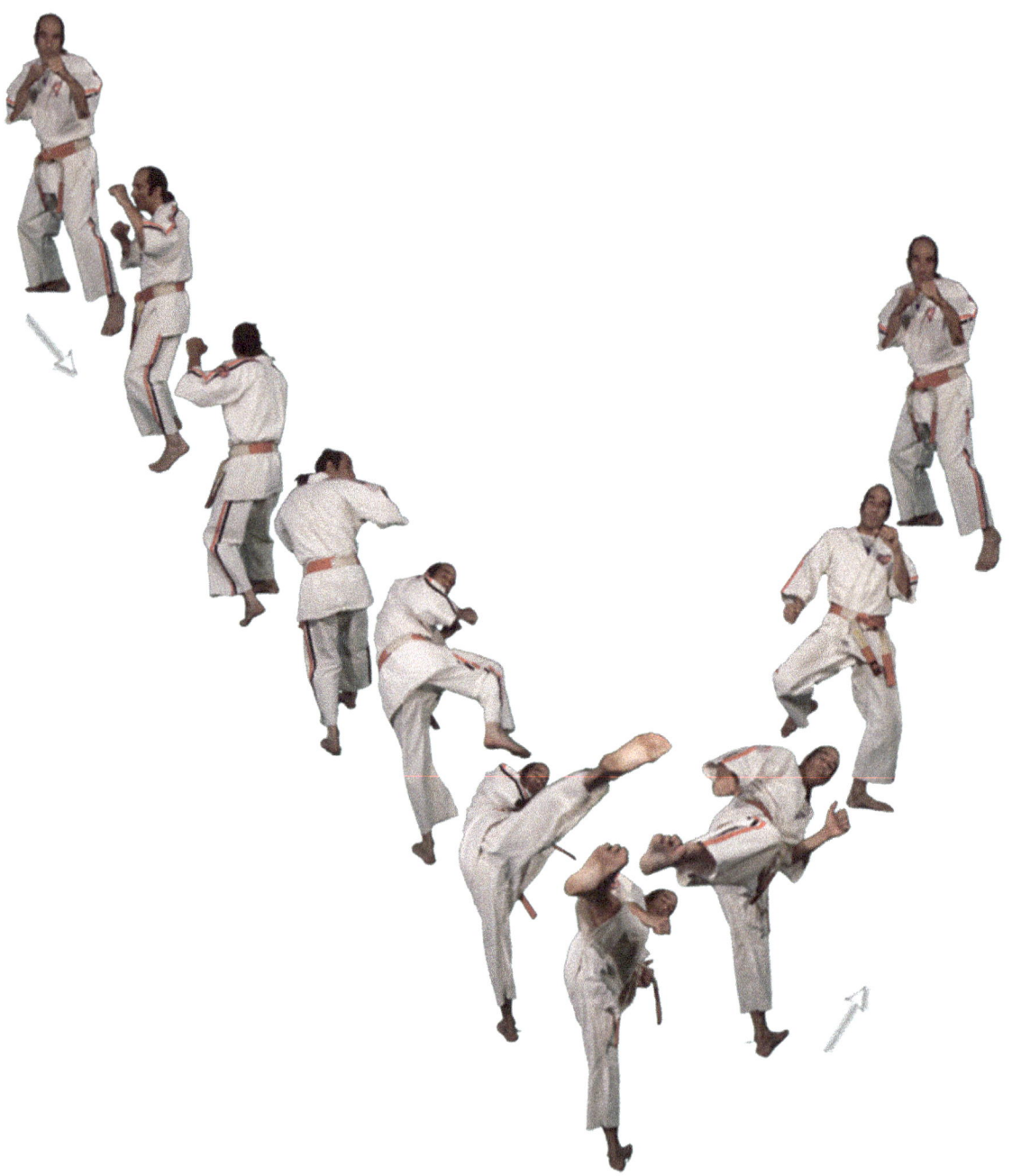

Figure 3.23: Illustrations of the Ushiro Mawashi Geri, from the front view.

USHIRO MAWASHI GERI: SIDE VIEW

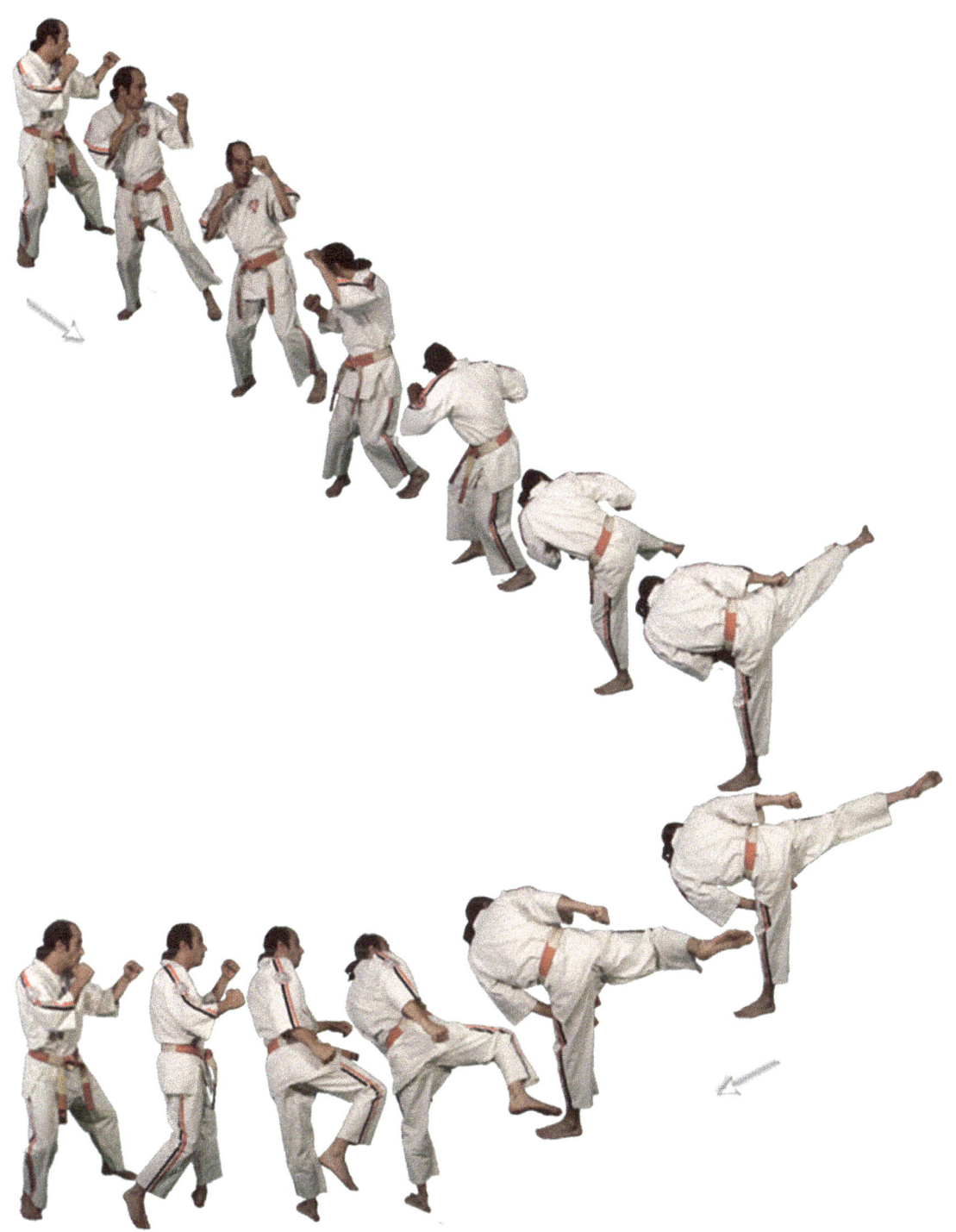

Figure 3.24: Illustrations of the Ushiro Mawashi Geri, from the side view.

3.4.3 STRIKING TECHNIQUES

Other than punching and kicking techniques, there are several other ways of striking that are very effective in real contact fighting situations and are referred to in Karate as Uchi Waza or Striking Techniques. They include _knee strikes, elbow strikes, knife hand strikes, hammer fist strikes and ridge hand strikes_. Like punching and kicking techniques, they all utilize the same principals of using the movement of the hips and shoulders and apply the weight of the whole body to drive the technique and maximize power and force. These striking techniques can be straight or circular just like punching or kicking techniques but can also be delivered downward and on angles that kicks and straight punches cannot access. Boxing techniques such as hooks, uppercuts and overhands have been developed to access these angles and can be interchanged with different striking techniques to accomplish similar results. The following section will outline the different Uchi Waza (striking techniques) and will also identify the techniques that can be substituted with similar effect.

A. Shuto Uchi (Knife Hand Strikes, Chopping techniques)

Probably the most recognizable of all techniques from Karate, the knife hand strike utilizes an open hand to strike with the palm side edge of the hand close to the wrist. This is known as the blade of the hand and utilizes about two inches of the edge of the hand from the wrist joint to about half way down the palm avoiding contact with the first knuckle joint of the little finger and the edge of the hand within at least one inch of that knuckle joint.

Contact can also be made safely with the bone knot of the wrist that is just below the traditional "blade" of the hand striking surface, however this doesn't change the mechanics of the techniques themselves. Knife hand strikes are particularly useful for attacking targets such as the side of the face and neck as they are delivered in a circular motion utilizing the twisting of the hips and shoulders to drive the blade of the hand in a circular motion to the target. Knife hand strikes are unique in that they can be delivered at a variety of different angles, such as downward, upward, or horizontal. As with all techniques, the limb delivering the technique must be kept relaxed right up until the point of contact where it is then tightened for impact.

Note: Most knife hand strikes share the same mechanics as back fist and hammer fist strikes and are basically the same with the difference being the contact point being utilized.

B. Ushiro Shuto Uchi (Back Chop with the Front Hand)

From a left fighting stance centered to the target, one must push off the right foot stepping forward with the left foot and place it in line with the left side of the opponent's body, keeping the centerline centered with the target. At the same time, the left hand must be brought close to the right side of the face with the arm and elbow joint lifted to that height protecting the face. One must start the rotation of the hips and shoulders clockwise towards the target and begin extending the edge of the hand towards the target by straightening the elbow. Contact must be made just before the technique reaches full extension and drives through the target reaching full extension, where the weight is on the left foot and the shoulders are turned to form a straight line from the edge of the hand to the back shoulder. The back shoulder must be pulled back to assist the turning of the hips and shoulders when executing the technique. This technique can be executed at different angles such as upward, downward, and horizontal by raising or lowering the starting position of the striking hand in relation to the target. In this way, one can strike on a downward angle by raising the starting position of the hand higher than the target. This would be useful against a shorter opponent to attack down onto the side of the neck or the collar bone or any situation where the target is lower than one's guard.

Likewise, one can strike with this technique at an upward angle by lowering the starting position of the hand below the height of the target. This can be useful against taller opponents and when attacking targets like the throat and the underside of the jawline. Of course, this technique can also be used horizontally to attach a target at the same height as the guard. A variation of this technique known as a back fist, can be done with a closed fist striking with the back part of the knuckles of the index and middle fingers. For this technique, the fist must be in a vertical position to the ground with the back of the knuckles pointing to the target. Perform all movements in reverse from a right fighting stance for a right back knife hand strike. See Figures 3.25 and 3.26 (below) and the accompanying video for illustration of Ushiro Shuto Uchi.

USHIRO SHUTO UCHI: FRONT VIEW

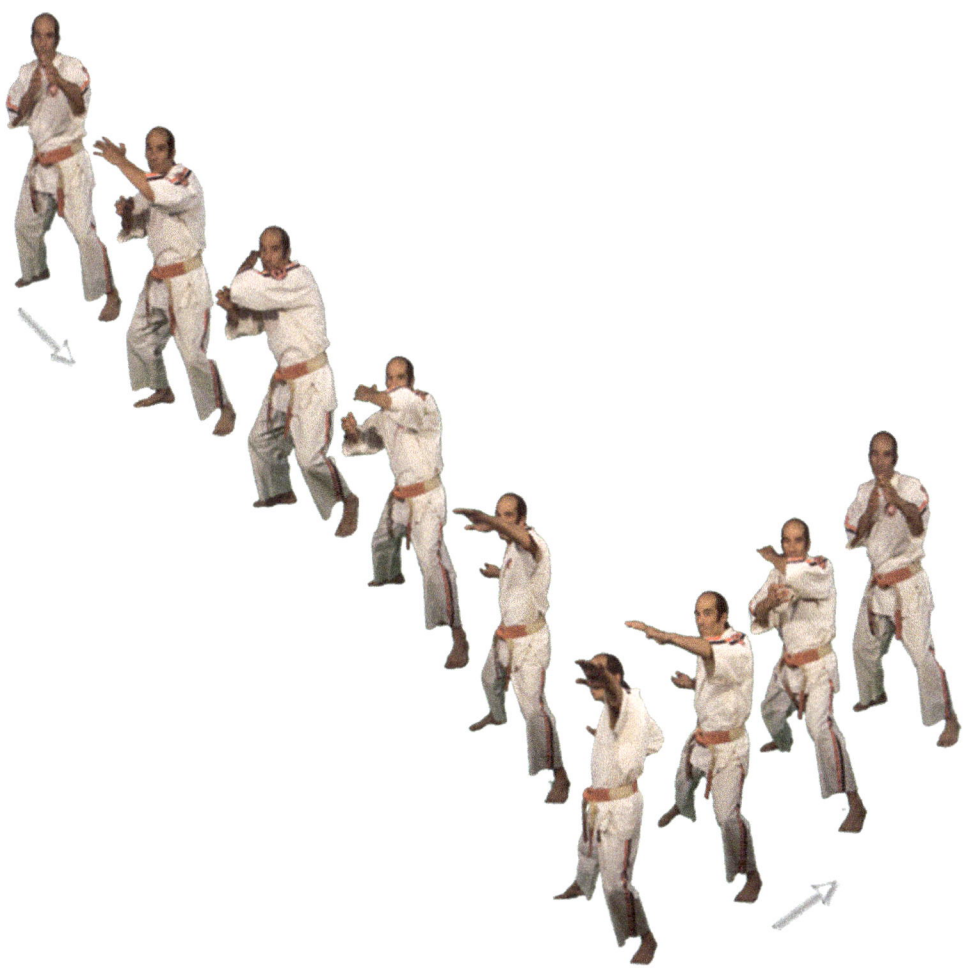

Figure 3.25: Illustrations of Ushiro Shuto Uchi, from the front view.

CHAPTER 3: PUNCHING, KICKING, AND STRIKING | 65

USHIRO SHUTO UCHI: SIDE VIEW

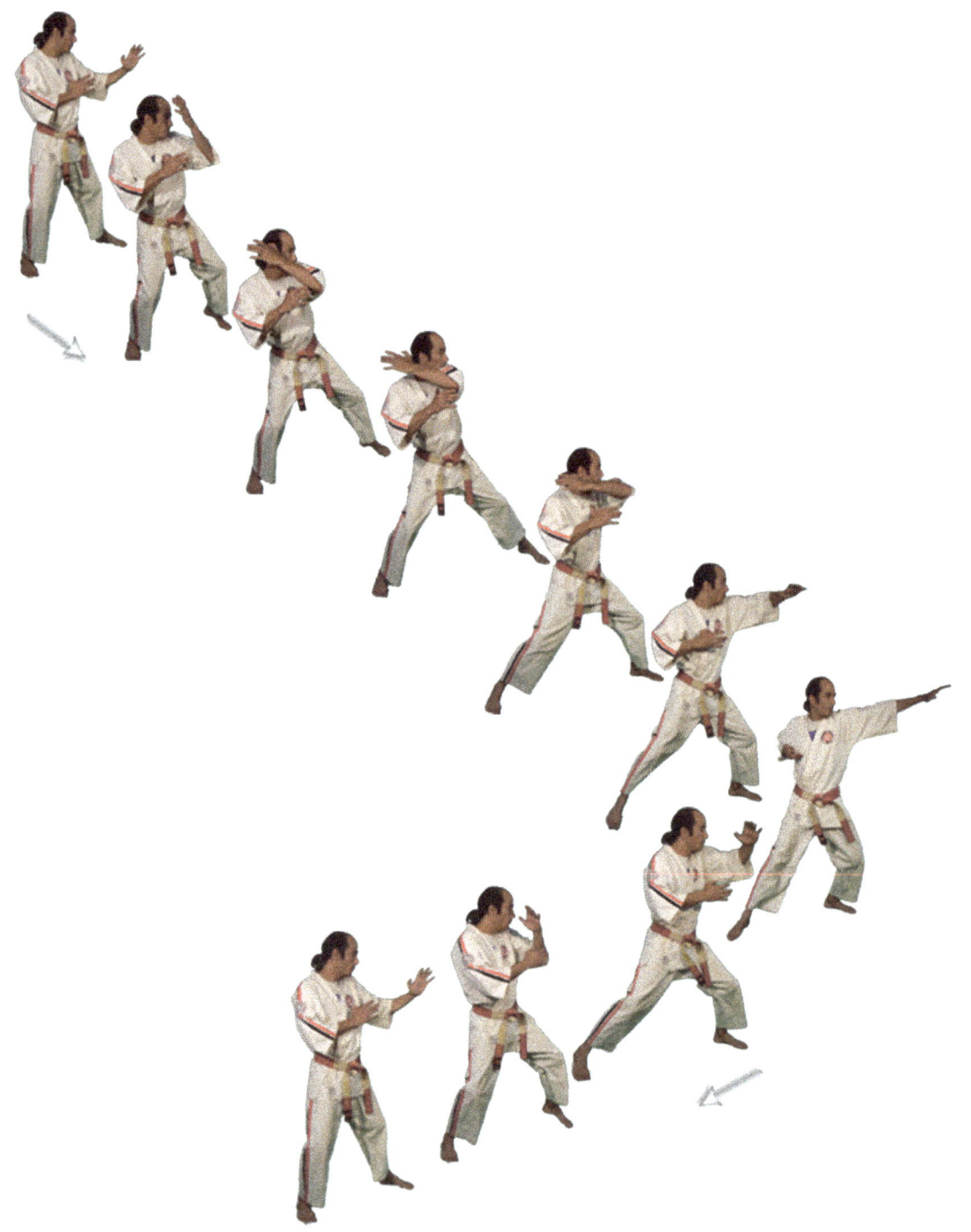

Figure 3.26: Illustrations of Ushiro Shuto Uchi, from the side view.

C. Mawari Ushiro Shuto Uchi (Turning/spinning Back knife hand strike or Back Fist)

This technique is widely used in professional fighting as it allows for a deceptive and powerful method of delivering a back chop or back fist with the back hand, which cannot utilize a back chop or back fist from a straight position. This technique is often used to follow up a circular technique by continuing the turning of the body and strikes as the back side comes around to become the front side. It utilizes the reverse lunging step as described in the previous chapter on stances and movement. This technique is also used in a defensive manner where the start of the technique can be disguised as turning to retreat from the opponent enticing an attack and catching them off-guard as they are about to attack.

From a left fighting stance centered to the target, one must slide the left foot to the right so that it crosses the body's center line. Next, one must push off the right foot and start rotating the body and head in a clockwise direction and step past the right foot close to the left foot as it moves towards the target and lands in striking distance slightly to the right of the target. The full turn must be completed before the right foot passes the left foot so that one is facing the direction of the target when entering the striking distance and not the back of one's head and body.

While making the turning motion, one must bring the right hand close to the left side of the face with the arm and elbow joint lifted to that height protecting the face. Then, one must begin extending the technique towards the target in the same way as described with Ushiro Shuto Uchi above. One must drop the body weight onto the right foot and extend the arm and shoulders into a straight line to the target focusing the body weight into the target to drive the technique. As above, contact can be made either with the edge/blade of the hand (Shuto Uchi) or with the back of the knuckles with a closed fist (Uraken Uchi).

Note: This type of back chop/fist is usually delivered on a horizontal plane. One must perform all movements in reverse from a right fighting stance for a left spinning Back knife hand strike. See Figure 3.27 (below) and the accompanying video for illustrations of Mawari Ushiro Shuto Uchi.

MAWARI USHIRO SHUTO UCHI

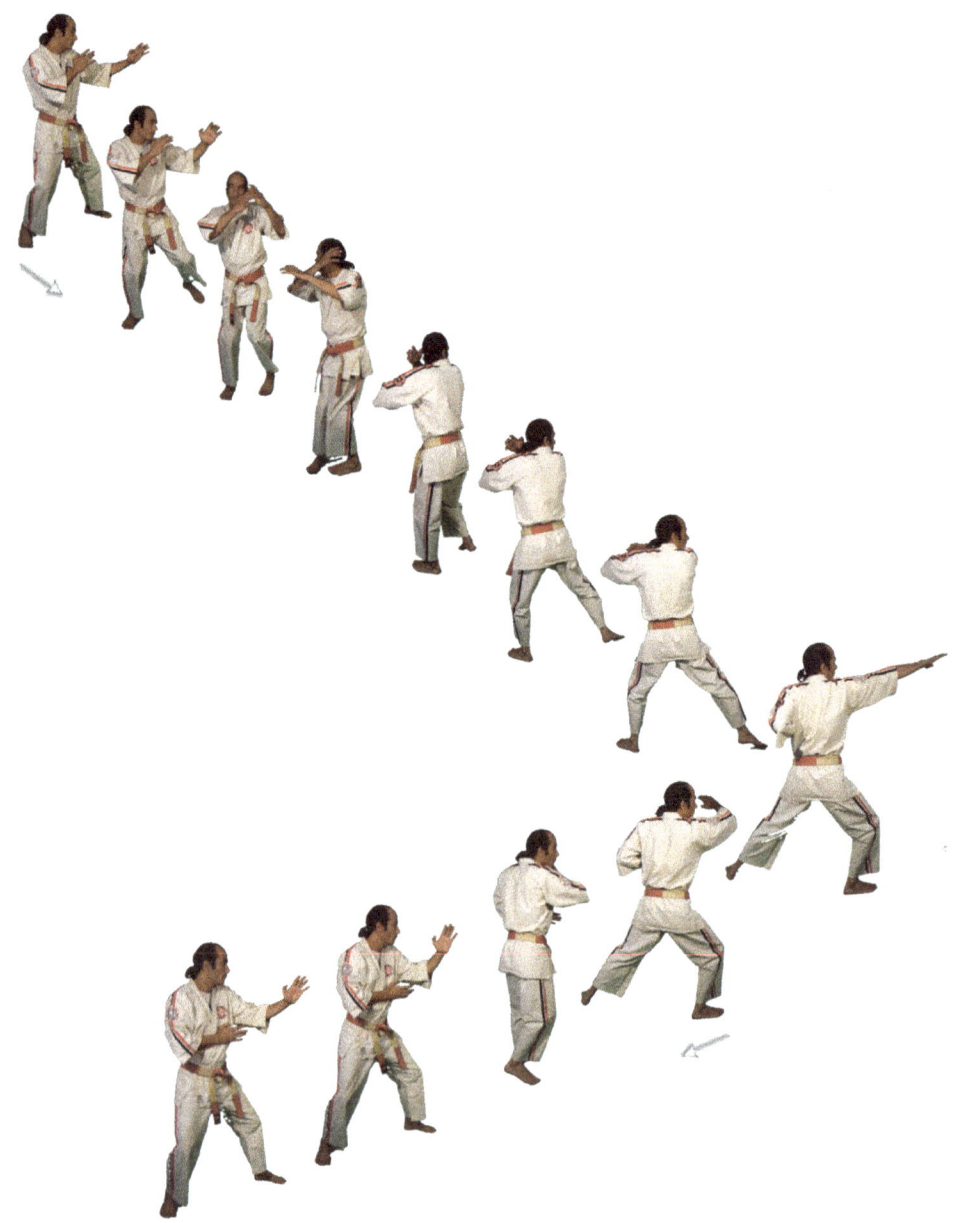

Figure 3.27: Illustrations of the Mawari Ushiro Shuto Uchi.

D. Mae Shuto Uchi (Front Knife Hand Strike, Front Chop)

The front knife hand strike is a very powerful chopping technique that is usually delivered on a downward angle much like chopping a tree with an axe or machete. It is one of the few strikes that can be delivered at this kind of downward and circular motion making it particularly useful when striking down to a fallen opponent, and also to deliver a strike at an unusual and sometimes awkward angle. The mechanics of this type of knife hand strike are often used with a closed fist utilizing the pad at the bottom of the fist, also known as a hammer fist strike. The hammer fist is used mostly down on the ground to attack a fallen opponent while the knife hand version of this technique is well suited for striking from a standing position to attach down onto the neck, collar, face, and head.

E. Oi Mae Shuto Uchi (Lunge Front Knife Hand Strike, Front Chop with the Front Hand)

From a left fighting stance centered to the target, one must push off the right foot stepping forward with the left foot and at the same time extending the right hand forward, down the center line to guard one's face. One must also bring the left hand back towards the left ear with the elbow bent and lifted up to shoulder height. This hand and arm position is similar to the position a baseball player would be in to successfully throw the baseball towards a far away target. In addition, one must place the left foot in line with the left side of the opponent and immediately begin rotating the hips and shoulders in a clockwise direction and begin extending the strike out to the target in a motion similar to how one would cast a fishing rod, forming an arc from over the head, out and down to the target, starting the arc left of the target on a downward angle in towards the target. This angle can be made larger or smaller as needed, making the technique either more horizontal or more vertical depending on the desired effect.

Contact can be made just prior to full extension in which the weight is just coming down on the front foot and the hips and shoulders are rotated until the hand, arm, and shoulders are in a straight line to the target. After the technique has been fully extended through the target, one must immediately pull back the left hand, extend the right hand to cover the face and push off the left foot and step back with the right foot into a left fighting stance. One must perform all movements in reverse from a right fighting stance for a right lunge front knife hand strike. See Figures 3.28 and 3.29 (below) and the accompanying video for illustrations of Oi Mae Shuto Uchi.

OI MAE SHUTO UCHI: FRONT VIEW

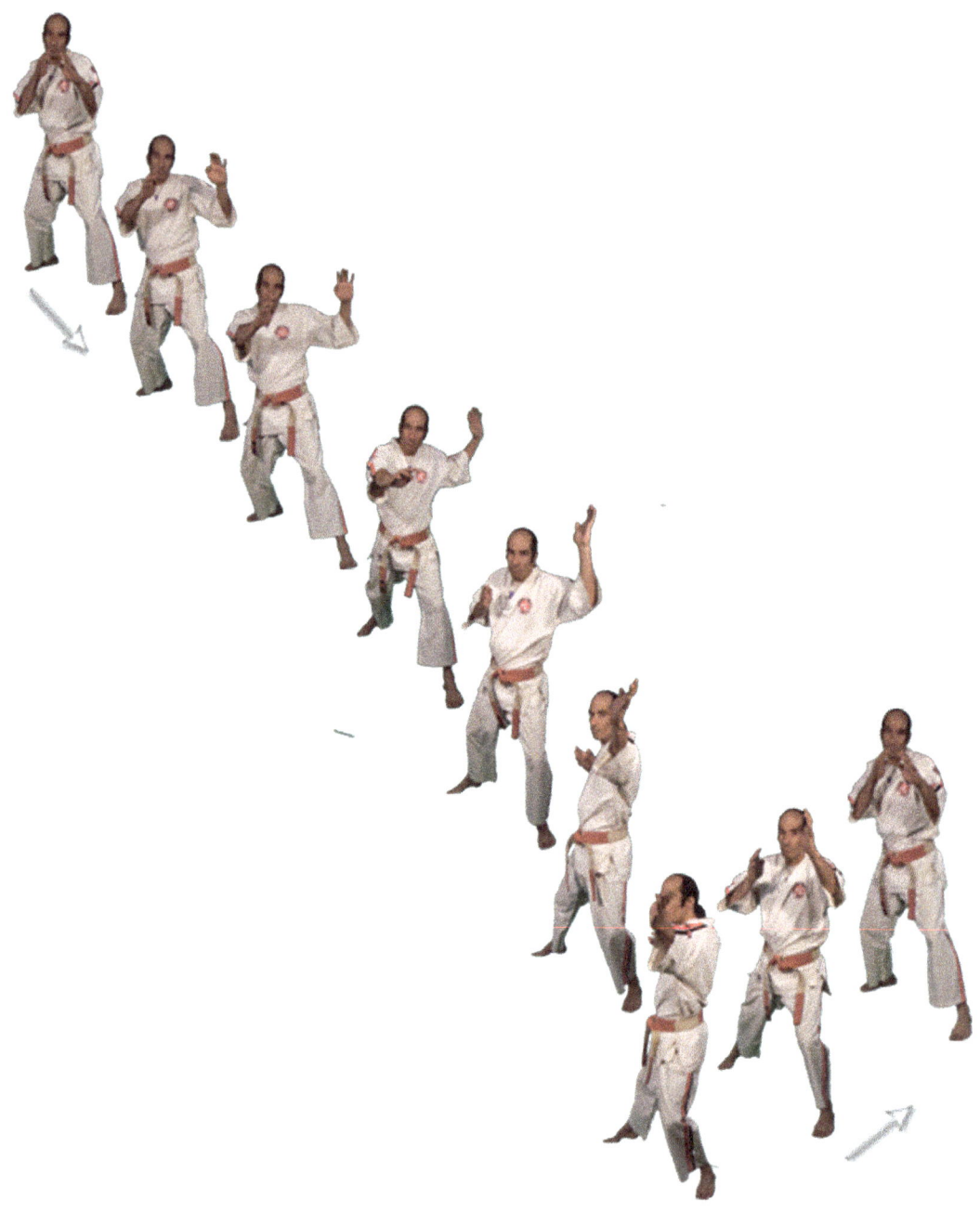

Figure 3.28: Illustrations of the Oi Mae Shuto Uchi, from the front view.

OI MAE SHUTO UCHI: SIDE VIEW

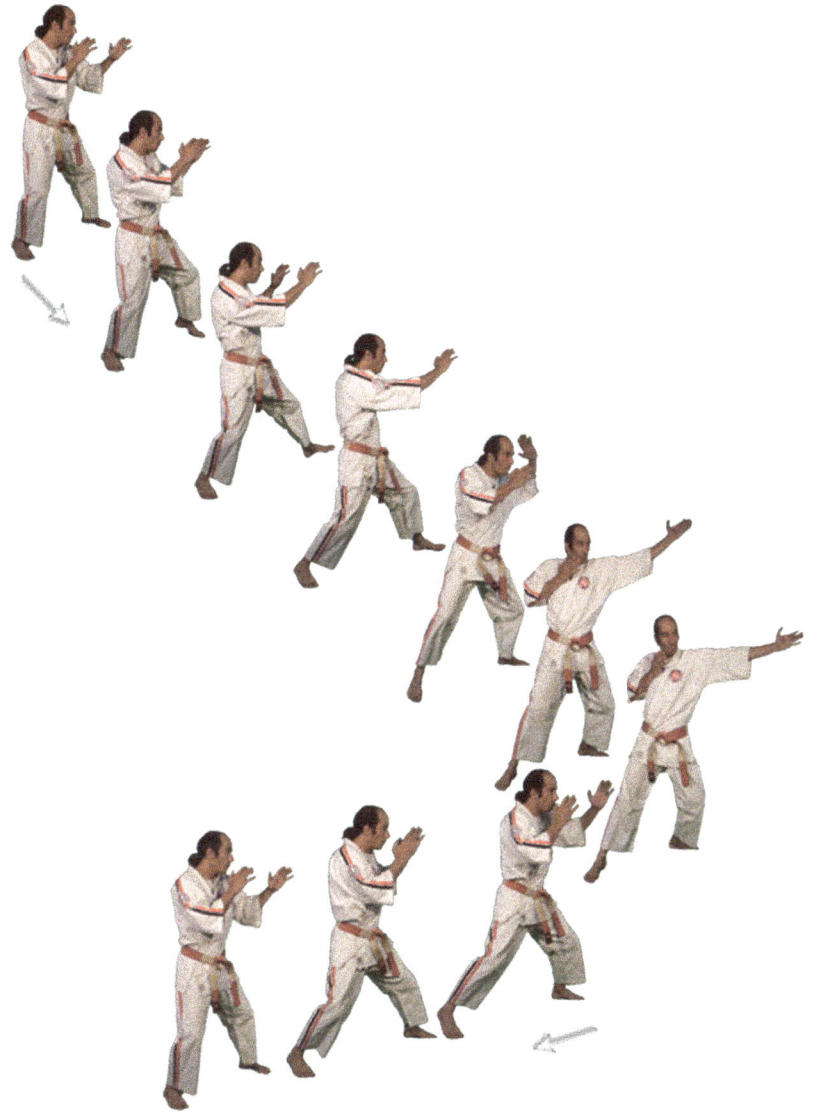

Figure 3.29: Illustrations of the Oi Mae Shuto Uchi, from the side view.

<u>F. Hineri Mae Shuto Uchi (Twist Front Knife Hand Strike, Front Chop with the Back Hand)</u>

From a left fighting stance centered to the target, one must push off the right foot, stepping forward with the left foot, and placing it at the necessary distance from the target keeping it in line (as with all techniques) with the left side of the opponent's body. One must also keep centered to the target and at the same time extend the left hand towards the target and simultaneously lift the right hand (i.e. striking hand) up towards the right ear with the elbow bent and lifted up to shoulder height or a little higher. As the left foot lands, one must immediately begin rotating/twisting the hips and shoulders in a counter clockwise direction and begin extending the technique out to the target in a motion. This is similar to how one would cast a fishing rod, forming an arc from over the head, out and down to the target and starting the arc right of the target on a downward angle in towards the target. This angle can be made larger or smaller as needed allowing for the technique to either be more horizontal or more vertical depending on the desired effect, however it is commonly used on a more vertical angle.

Contact must be made just prior to full extension in which the weight is on the front foot and the hips and shoulders are rotated until the striking hand, arm, and shoulders are in a straight line to the target. After the technique has been fully extended through the target, one must immediately pull back the right hand and extend the left hand to cover the face and push off the left foot stepping back with the right foot into a left fighting stance. One must perform all movements in reverse from a right fighting stance for a left twist front knife hand strike. See Figures 3.30 and 3.31 (below) and the accompanying video for illustrations of Hineri Mae Shuto Uchi.

HINERI MAE SHUTO UCHI: FRONT VIEW

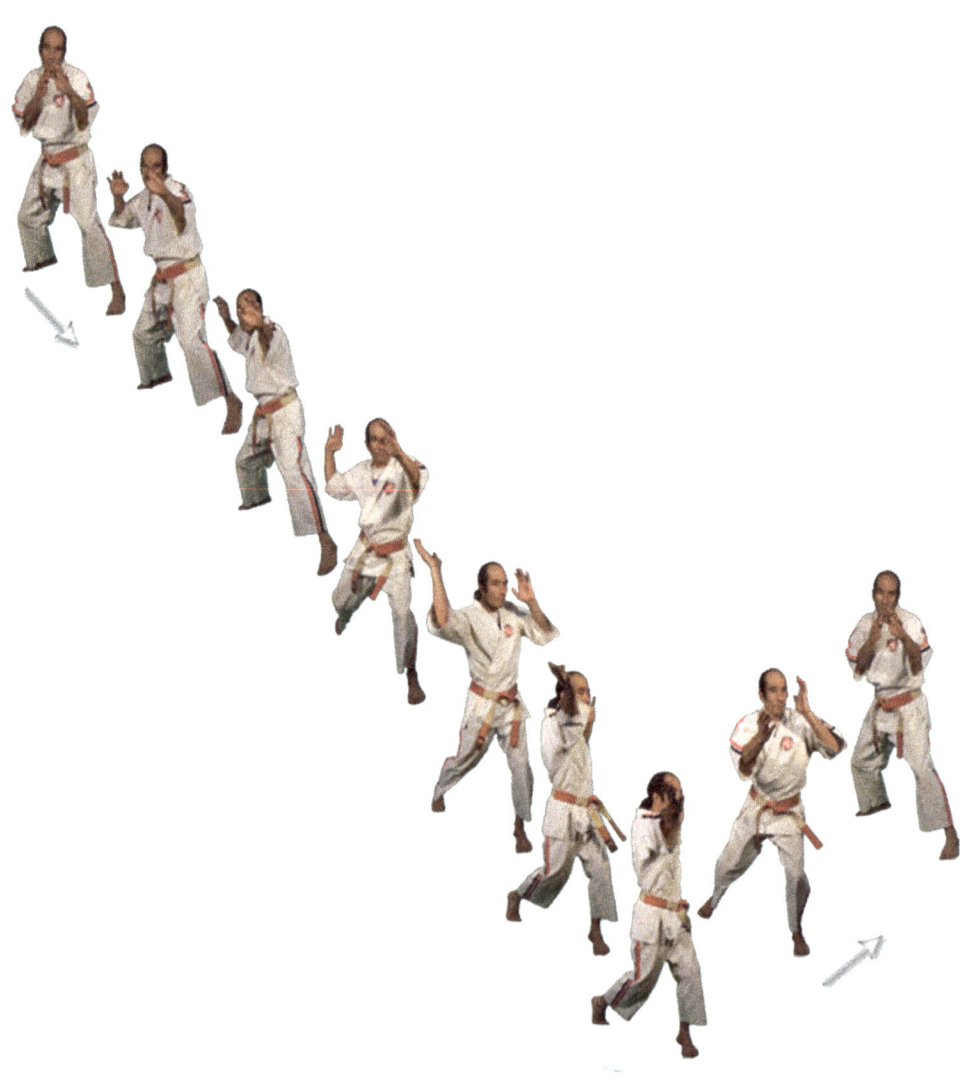

Figure 3.30: Illustrations of Hineri Mae Shuto Uchi, from the front view.

HINERI MAE SHUTO UCHI: SIDE VIEW

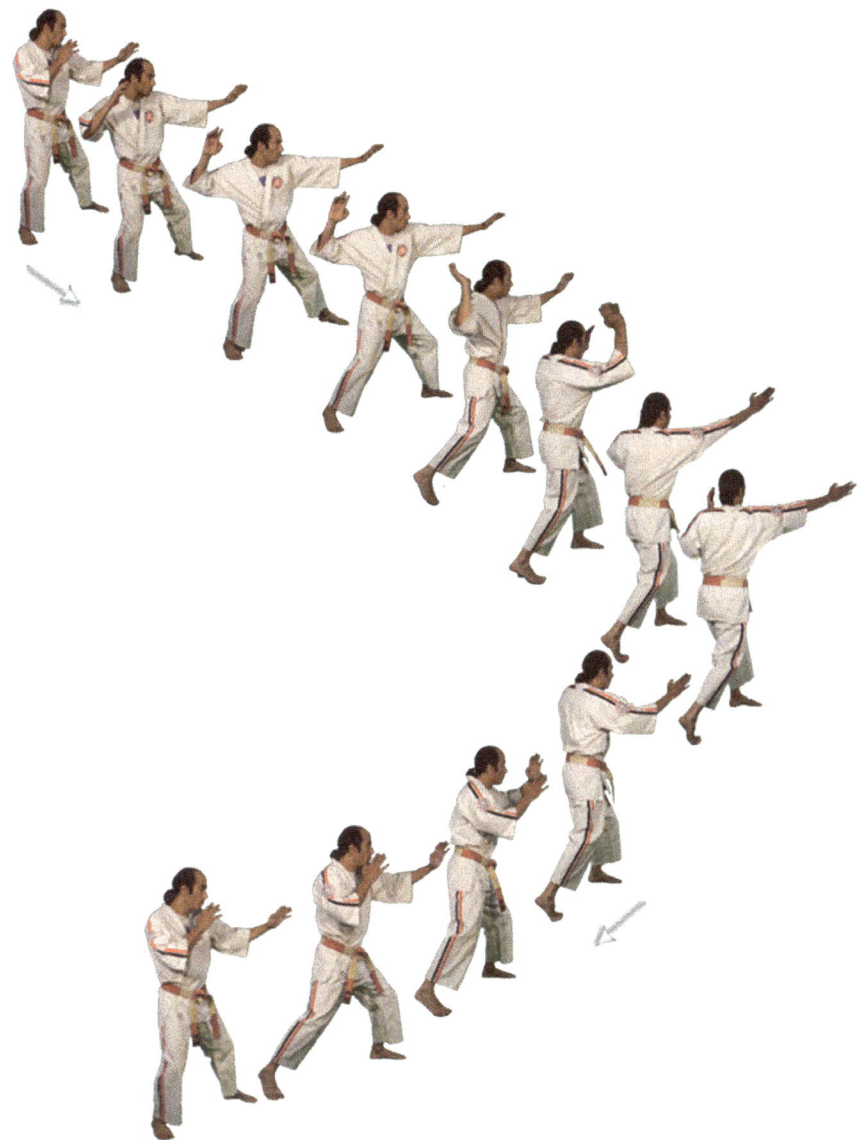

Figure 3.31: Illustrations of Hineri Mae Shuto Uchi, from the side view.

G. Haito Uchi and Soto Kentsui Uchi (Ridge hand and outside hammer fist)

The ridge hand and the outside hammer fist are both techniques where contact is made with the base of the knuckle joint of the thumb and the side of the first knuckle joint of the index finger and can also utilize the side of the wrist bone and the bottom of the forearm. The only difference with these two techniques is that the ridge hand is delivered with an open hand with the thumb tucked into the palm and the outside hammer is delivered with a closed fist. (See fig for illustration of hand position and striking points for ridge hand and outside hammer fist). It is delivered in a circular motion to the target and is driven by a twisting of the hips and shoulders and can look similar to the "clothes line" technique used in sports like American football however it is not delivered with a straight arm but rather thrown straight out and then around in a whipping motion driven by the twisting of the hips. The ridge hand is mainly used to attack targets such as the side of the face, the Jaw line and the side of the neck and the reverse hammer fist is mainly used to attack body targets. While this technique can be executed with both the lead hand and the back hand it is mainly used with the back hand.

H. Hineri Haito/Soto Kentsui Uchi (Twist Ridge Hand/Outside Hammer Fist Strike)

From a Left fighting stance centered to the target, push off the right leg stepping forward and slightly left of the target with the left foot, placing it at the correct distance from the target to deliver the technique. Begin Twisting/rotating the hips and shoulders in a counter clockwise direction and then begin extending the right hand straight out in a direction just to the right of the target and bring it into the target as the right hip and shoulder come in line with the target line. When the hand reaches about 2/3 of the way out, turn the hand counter clockwise until the palm of the hand is pointing downward and the ridge of the hand is focused to the target, it is then circled into the target for the last 1/3 of the technique. The delivery of this technique should be thrown in a smooth whipping motion driven by the rotation of the hips and shoulders. The technique is fully extended when the shoulders form a straight line with the striking arm and the target, however it is important to keep a slight bend in the elbow of the striking arm to avoid any injury to the elbow joint. The reverse hammer fist is executed the same way except the fist is closed at the moment of contact focusing the contact as described above for reverse hammer fist. After full extension immediately pull back the hand hips and shoulders and push off the left foot stepping back with the right foot into a left fighting stance. Perform all movements in reverse from a right fighting stance for a left twist ridge hand/reverse hammer fist strike. See Figure 3.32 on next page and video for illustration of Hineri Haito/Soto Kentsui Uchi.

HINERI HAITO/ SOTO KENTSUI UCHI: FRONT AND SIDE VIEW

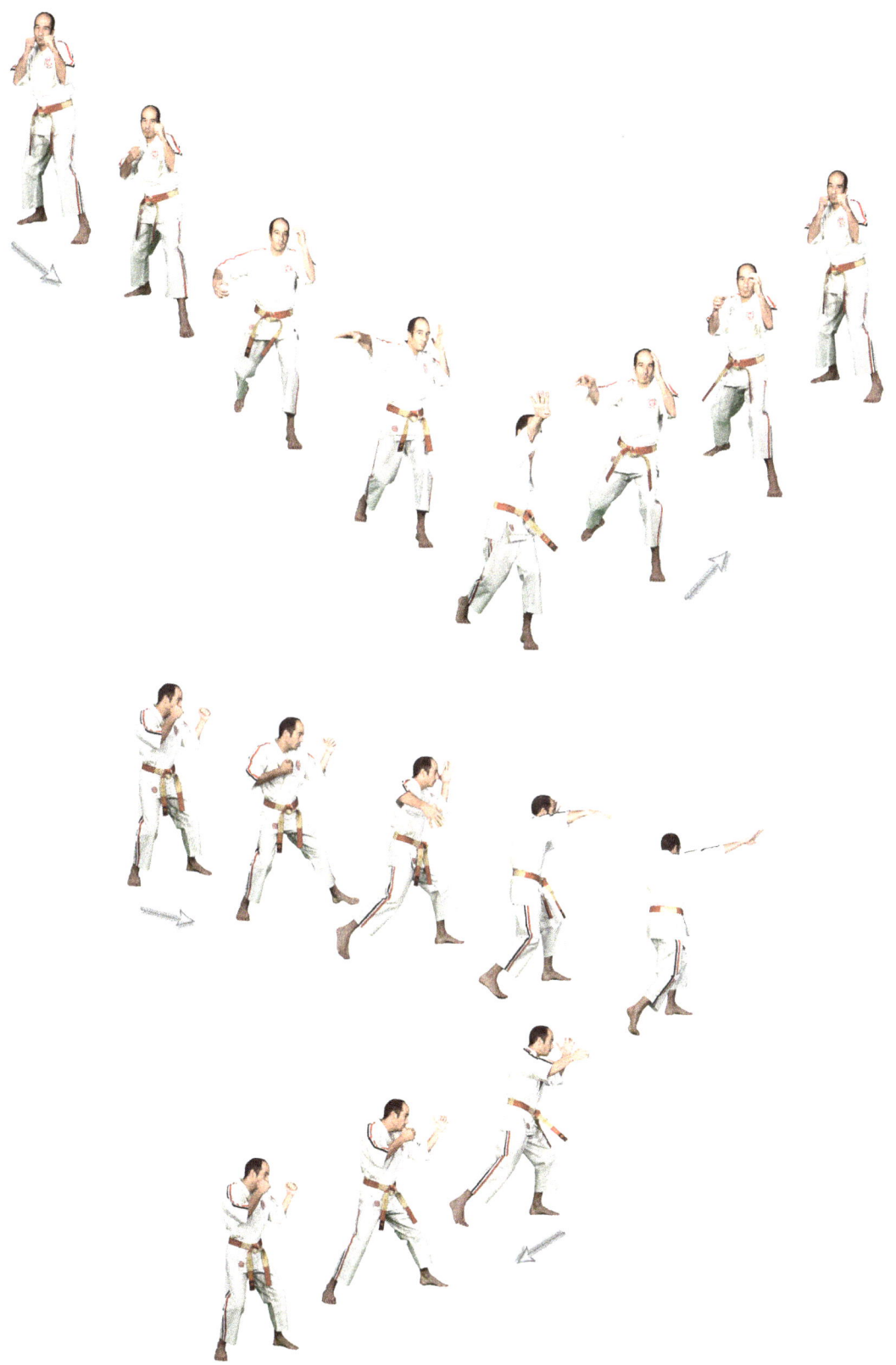

Figure 3.32: Illustrations of Hineri Haito/Soto Kentsni Uchi, from the front and side views.

I. Hiza Geri and Empi Uchi (Knee and Elbow Strikes)

Knee and elbow strikes are very popular and widely used techniques. They are very important because they are by nature very close range techniques and are used when the opponent is too close to make use of regular kicking and punching techniques, oftentimes in a clinch or grabbing scenario. These close range techniques are particularly useful because they can be delivered straight to the target, upwards, circular, and at multiple angles. In many cases, these techniques are delivered while holding the opponent with one or both hands thus, making it difficult for the opponent to escape or create distance.

Elbow techniques are generally focused to the target's head while knees are mostly focused at body targets. However, knees can also be used on the target's head, particularly when pulling down on the opponent's head when in a clinching or grappling situation. The mechanics used to generate power with these techniques are the same as with all other techniques. They use the twisting or thrusting of the hips to drive the technique with the weight of the body to maximize power.

J. Mae Empi Uchi (Straight Elbow Techniques)

These elbow techniques share the same movement and mechanics as the straight punching techniques however, they are delivered at about half the distance. Contact is made not with the elbow joint itself but with the part of the forearm that is just below the elbow joint. This type of elbow strike can be delivered from a fighting stance or while grabbing/holding the opponent with the non-striking hand and pulling into the strike. Another version of the straight elbow is the upward elbow, known as the Age Empi Uchi which is quite similar. However, it requires the striking elbow to be delivered upwards by pulling the hand right back to the ear while lifting the elbow higher than the target, generally under the chin or the face if it is facing downward.

K. Oi Mae Empi Uchi (Lunge Straight Elbow Strike, Straight Elbow with the Front Arm)

From a left fighting stance centered to the target, one must push off the right foot stepping forward with the left foot and place it in line with the left side of the opponent's body, while keeping one's centerline centered with the target. One must start rotating the hips and shoulders clockwise towards the target. The forearm must then be extended into the target with the arm bent at approximately 80-90 degrees, tightening on contact and forming a straight line from the elbow to the back shoulder.

For maximum power to be achieved, contact should be timed so that it occurs just before one's body weight settles on their left foot. After contact is made and extension is achieved, the technique must be immediately relaxed and pulled back to its starting position by retracting the hips and shoulders back to their starting position, finishing in the left fighting stance. For the upward elbow strike, the hand of the striking arm must be pulled right back to the ear and the strike must be delivered upward while slightly raising the body weight. One must perform all movements in reverse from a right fighting stance for a right lunge straight elbow strike. See Figures 3.33 and 3.34 and the accompanying video for illustrations of Oi Empi Uchi and Age Empi Uchi.

OI MAE EMPI UCHI: SIDE VIEW

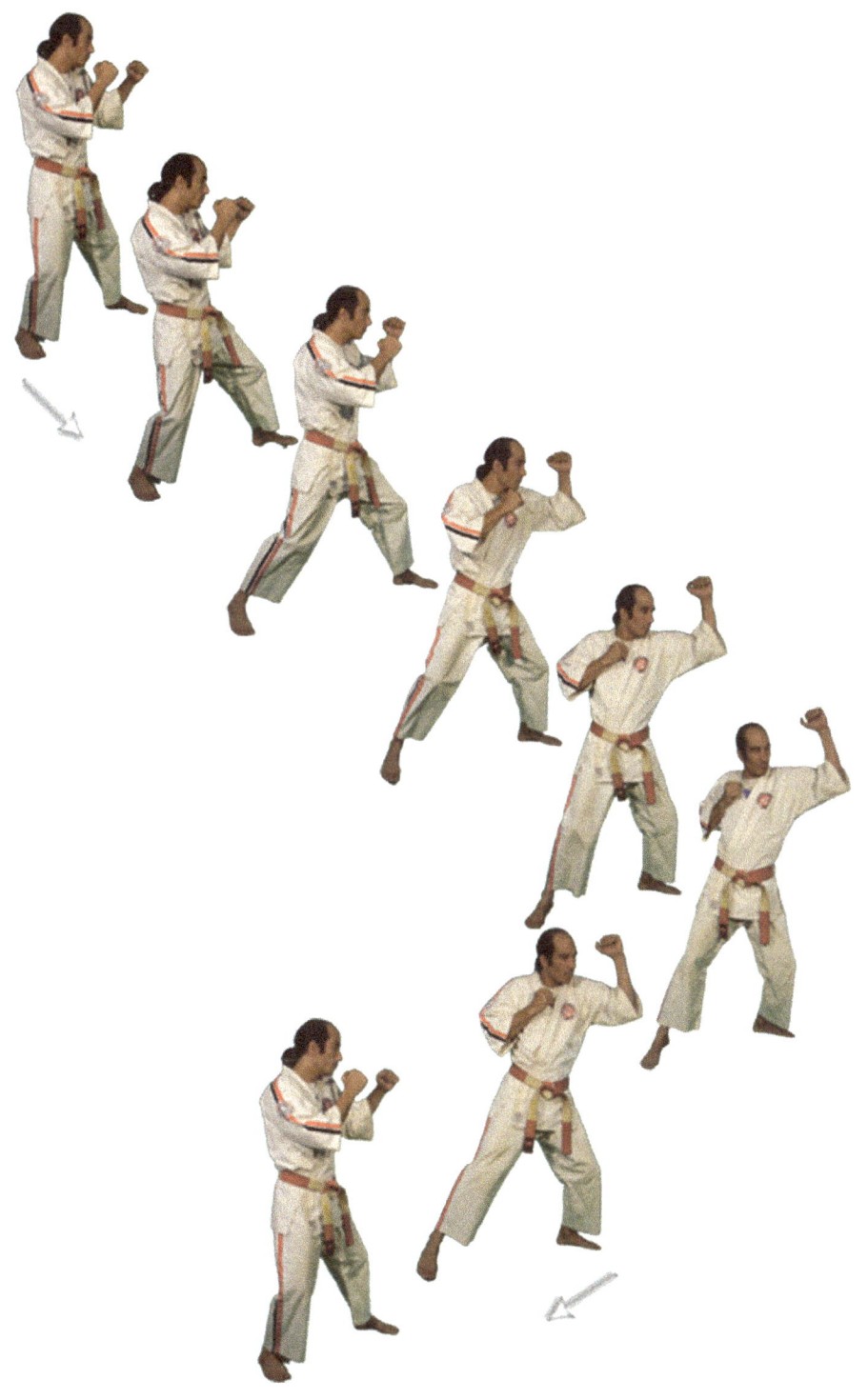

Figure 3.33: Illustrations of the Oi Mae Empi Uchi, from the side view.

OI MAE EMPI UCHI: FRONT VIEW

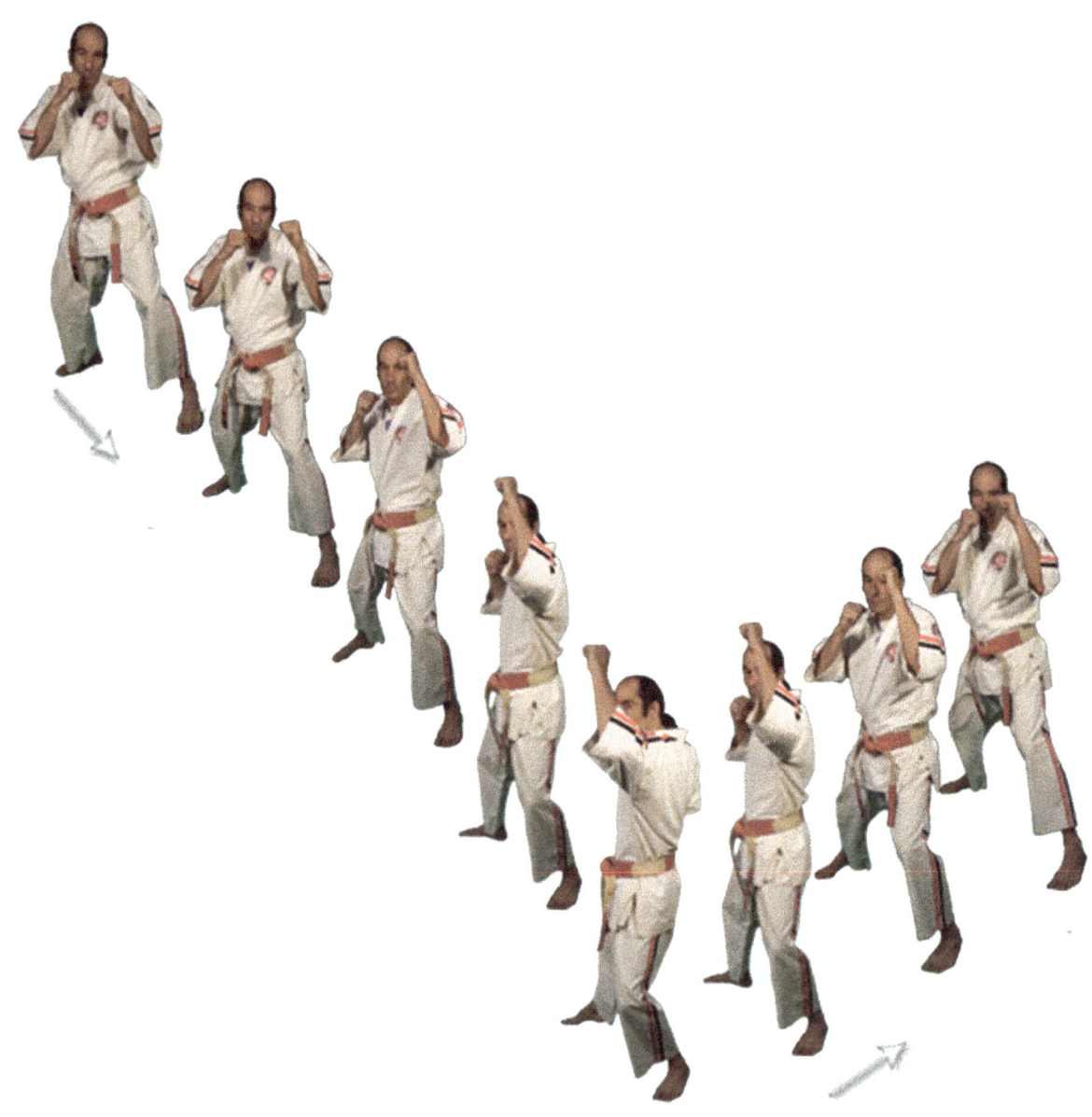

Figure 3.34: Illustrations of the Oi Mae Empi Uchi, from the front view.

L. Hineri Mae Empi Uchi (Twist Straight Elbow Strike, Straight Elbow with the Back Hand)

From a left fighting stance centered to the target, one must push off the right foot, stepping forward with the left foot in line with the opponent's left side while dropping the body weight onto the left foot. One must immediately start rotating the hips and shoulders counter clockwise towards the target. The right forearm is then extended into the target, with the arm bent at approximately 80-90 degrees tightening on contact and forming a straight line from the right elbow to the left shoulder. Power can be maximized by timing the contact at the moment one's body weight is settled on the left foot. After contact is made and extension is achieved, the arm must be immediately relaxed and pulled back to its starting position by retracting the hips and shoulders back to their starting position, thereby finishing in a balanced fighting stance. One must perform all movements in reverse from a right fighting stance for a left twist straight elbow strike. See Figures 3.35 and 3.36 (below) and video for illustration of Hineri Empi Uchi and Age Empi Uchi.

HINERI MAE EMPI UCHI: FRONT VIEW

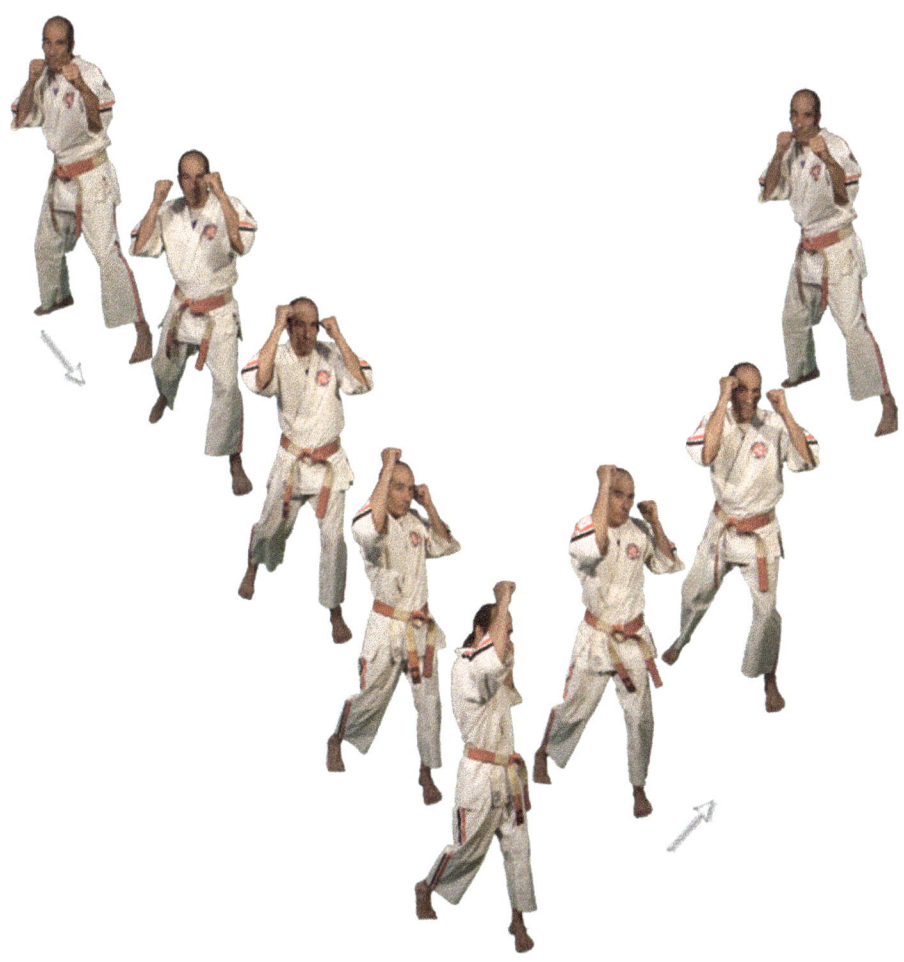

Figure 3.35: Illustrations of Hineri Mae Empi Uchi, from the front view.

HINERI MAE EMPI UCHI: SIDE VIEW

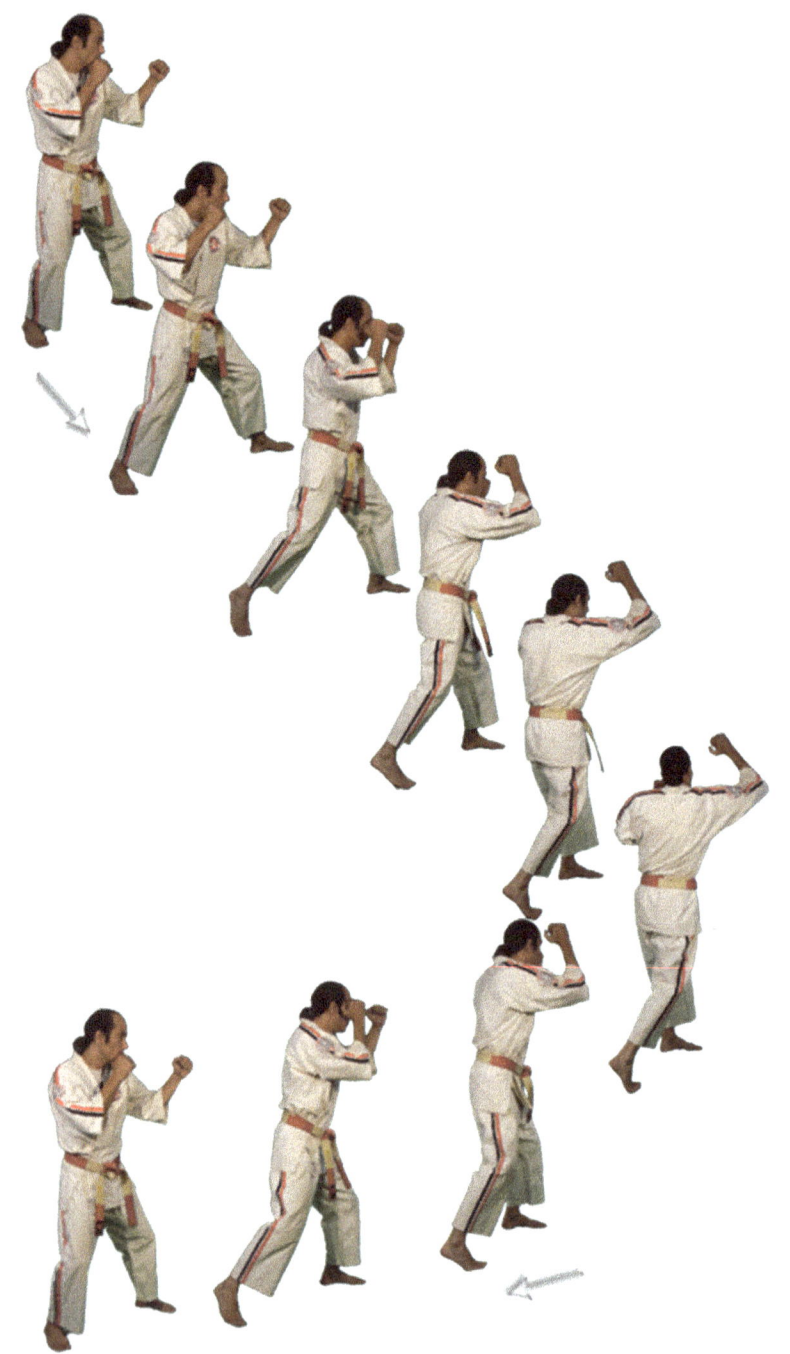

Figure 3.36: Illustrations of Hineri Mae Empi Uchi, from the side view.

M. Mawashi Empi Uchi (Roundhouse Elbow Strike)

The roundhouse elbow strike is a very popular and useful technique as the knife hand strikes with an angle of delivery that can be altered to suit the situation. These strikes share similar body mechanics as the front knife hand strike. With this elbow strike, the hand is pulled into the body as the forearm is swung in a circular motion towards the target again driven by the rotation of the hips and shoulders.

N. Oi Mawashi Empi Uchi (Lunge Roundhouse Elbow Strike, Roundhouse Elbow with the Front Arm)

From a left fighting stance centered to the target, one must push off the right foot stepping forward with the left foot and at the same time lifting the left elbow to the height of the target with the palm of the hand facing down to the ground. Then, one must place the left foot in line with the left side of the opponent and immediately begin rotating the hips and shoulders in a clockwise direction, driving the forearm in a circular motion into the target. Contact must be made just prior to full extension in which the weight is just coming down on the front foot and the hips and shoulders are rotated until the elbow, arm, and shoulders are in a straight line to the target. After the technique has been fully extended through the target, one must immediately retract the hips and shoulders, returning to guard position and push off the left foot stepping back with the right foot into a left fighting stance. One must perform all movements in reverse from a right fighting stance for a right lunge roundhouse elbow strike. See Figures 3.37 and 3.38 below and video for illustration of Oi Mawashi Empi Uchi.

OI MAWASHI EMPI UCHI: FRONT VIEW

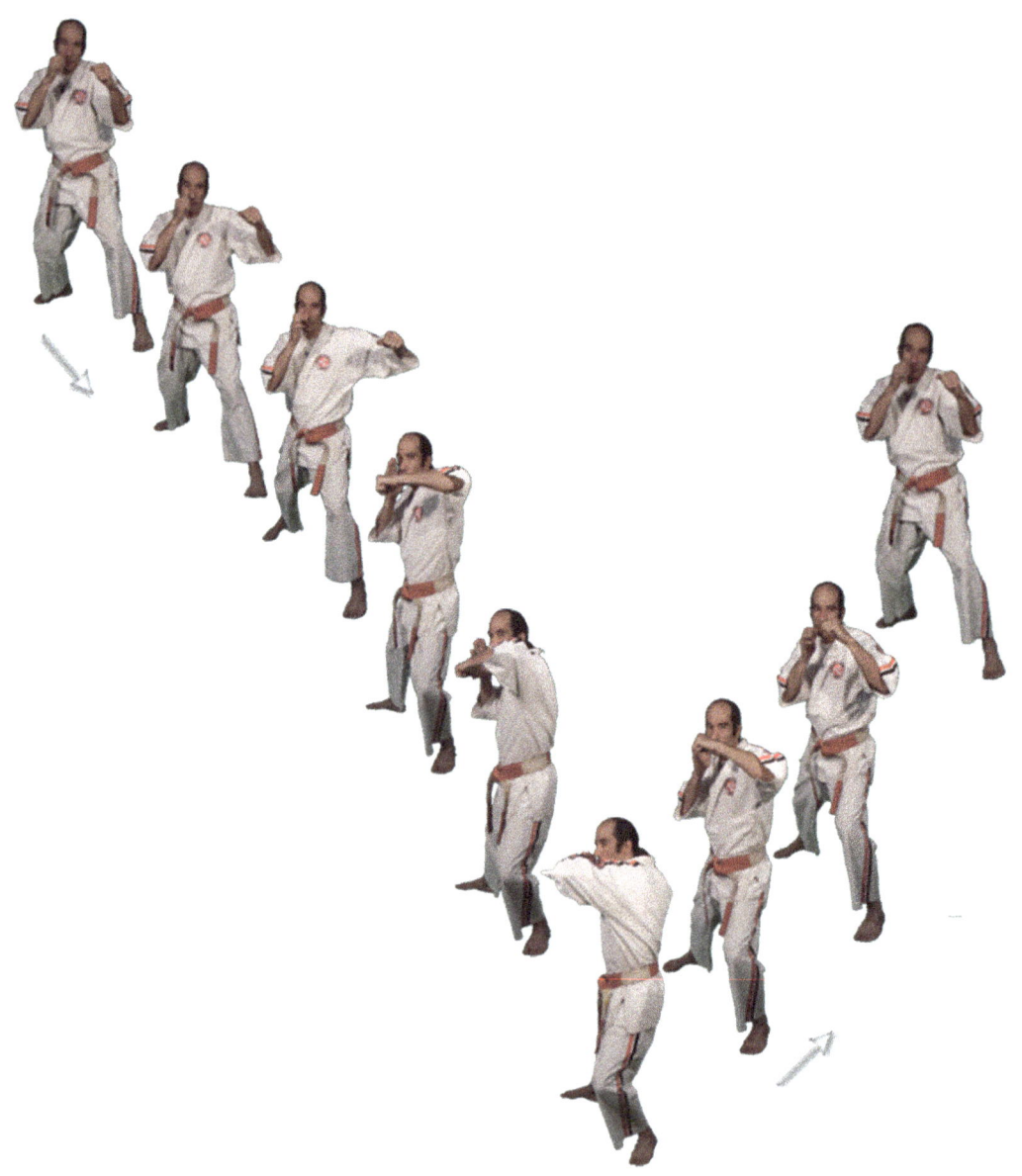

Figure 3.37: Illustrations of Oi Mawashi Empi Uchi, from the front view.

OI MAWASHI EMPI UCHI: SIDE VIEW

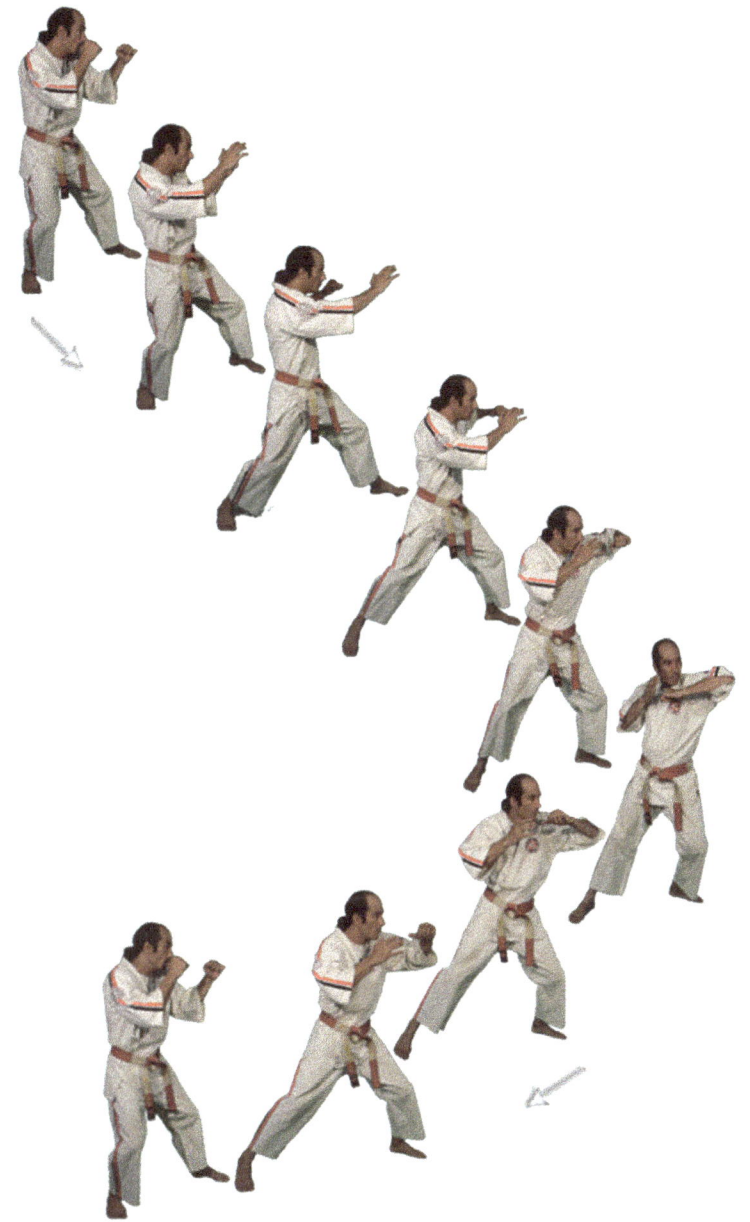

Figure 3.38: Illustrations of Oi Mawashi Empi Uchi, from the side view.

O. Hineri Mawashi Empi Uchi (Twist Roundhouse Elbow Strike, Roundhouse Elbow Strike with the Back Arm)

From a left fighting stance centered to the target, one must push off the right foot stepping forward with the left foot and place it at the necessary distance from the target keeping it in line (as with all techniques) with the left side of the opponent's body. At the same time, one must lift the right elbow to the height of the target with the palm of the hand facing down to the ground. As the left foot lands, immediately begin rotating/twisting the hips and shoulders in a counter clockwise direction driving the forearm in a circular motion into the target.

Contact can be made just prior to full extension in which the weight is on the front foot and the hips and shoulders must be rotated until the elbow, arm, and shoulders are in a straight line to the target. After the technique has been fully extended through the target, one must immediately retract the hips and shoulders returning to guard position and push off the left foot, stepping back with the right foot into a left fighting stance. One must perform all movements in reverse from a right fighting stance for a left twist roundhouse elbow strike. See Figures 3.39 and 3.40 (below) and video for illustration of Hineri Mawashi Empi Uchi.

HINERI MAWASHI EMPI UCHI: FRONT VIEW

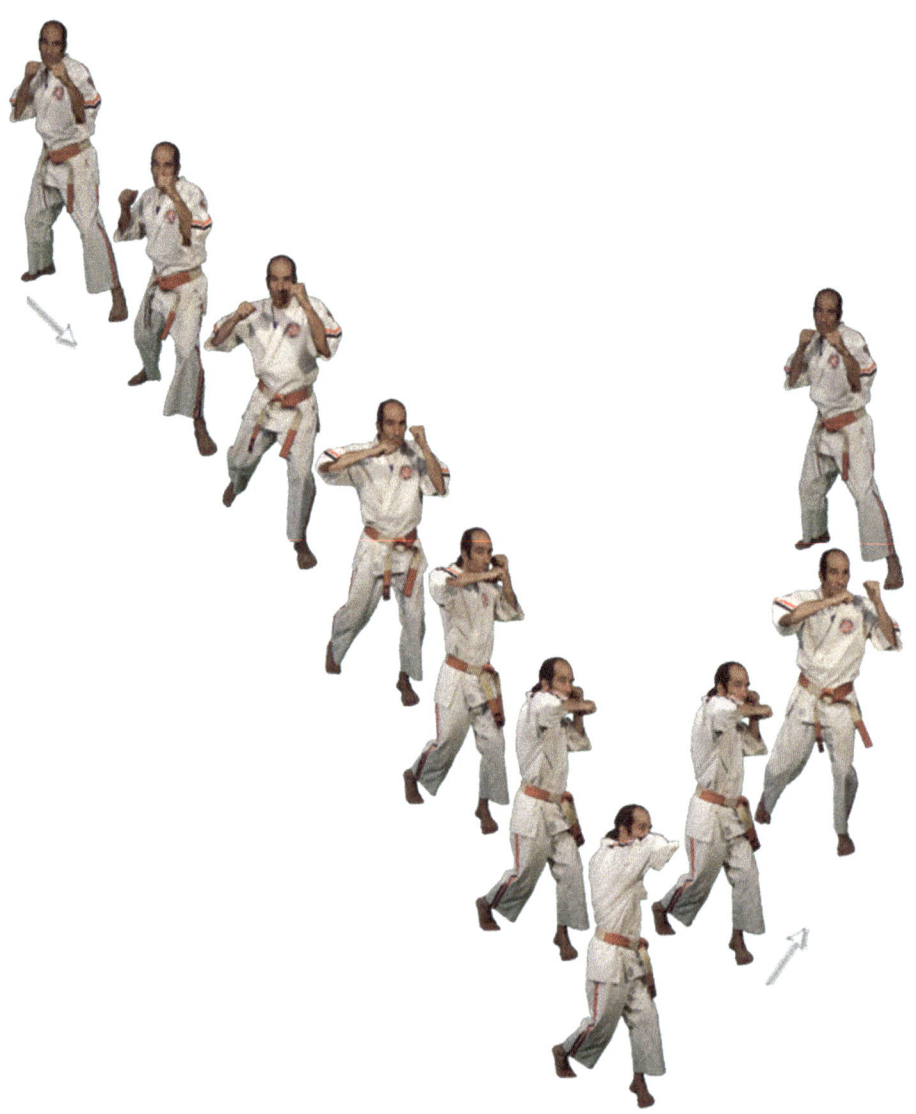

Figure 3.39: Illustrations of Hineri Mawashi Empi Uchi, from the front view.

HINERI MAWASHI EMPI UCHI: SIDE VIEW

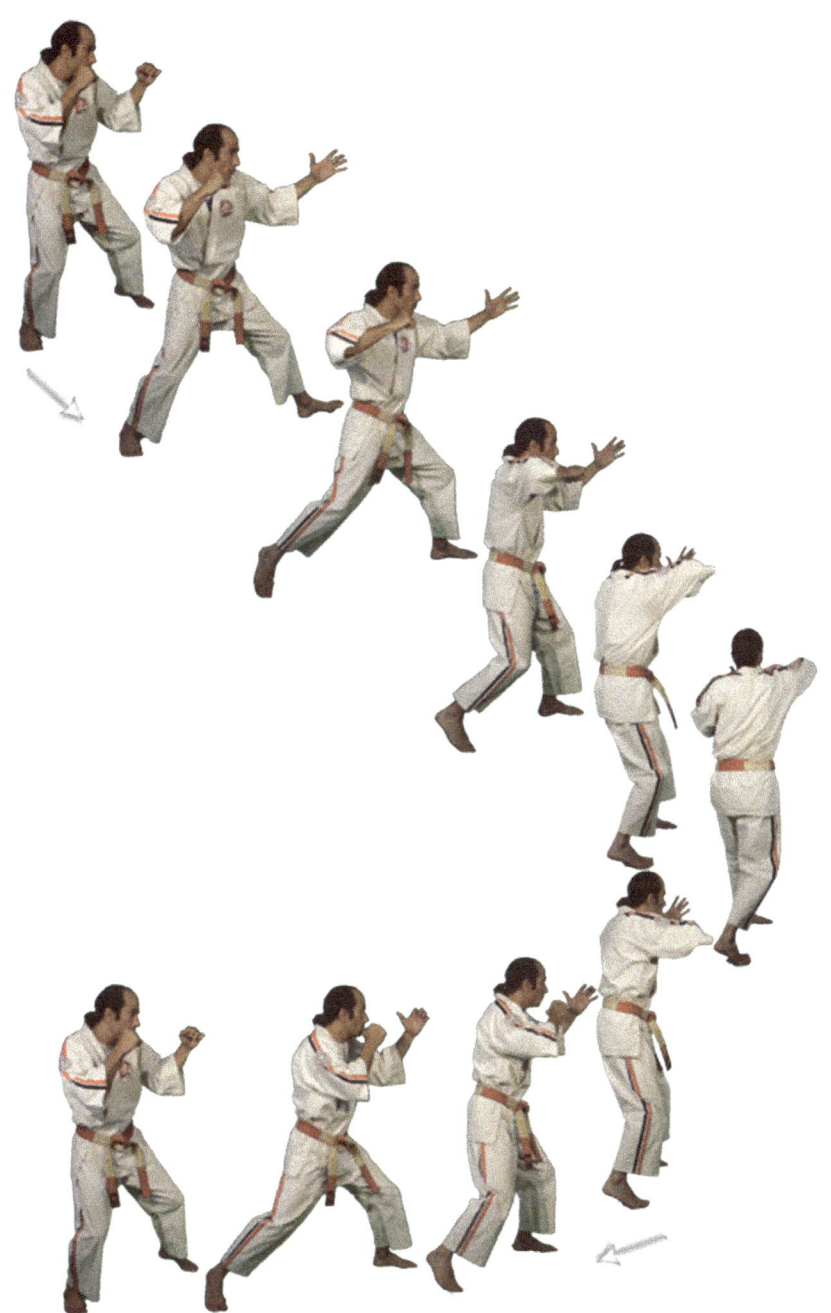

Figure 3.40: Illustrations of Hineri Mawashi Empi Uchi, from the side view.

P. Otoshi Empi Uchi (Downward Elbow Strikes)

Unlike the straight and roundhouse elbows the downward elbow utilizes the back side of the elbow above the elbow joint. It is commonly used in grappling situations on the ground but can be used in standing striking situations to strike down on the top of the head and face.

Q. *Oi Otoshi Empi Uchi (Downward Elbow with the Front Arm)*

From a left fighting stance centered to the target, one must push off the right foot stepping forward with the left foot and at the same time lifting the left elbow above the height of the target with the palm of the hand above the left ear and the elbow fully bent. One must also place the left foot in line with the left side of the opponent and slightly rotate the hips and shoulders in a clockwise direction, then immediately bring the elbow down onto the target making contact with the back of the arm close to the elbow joint (the point of the elbow can also be used when coming down on facial targets) and dropping the center of gravity to drive the strike downward with the weight of the body. On contact, the elbow is tightened along with the muscles and tendons of the hand and wrist. After making contact, one must push off the left foot stepping back into a left fighting stance. One must perform all movements in reverse from a right fighting stance for a right lunge downward elbow strike. See Figures 3.42 and 3.43 (below) and video for illustration of Oi Otoshi Empi Uchi.

OI OTOSHI EMPI UCHI: FRONT VIEW

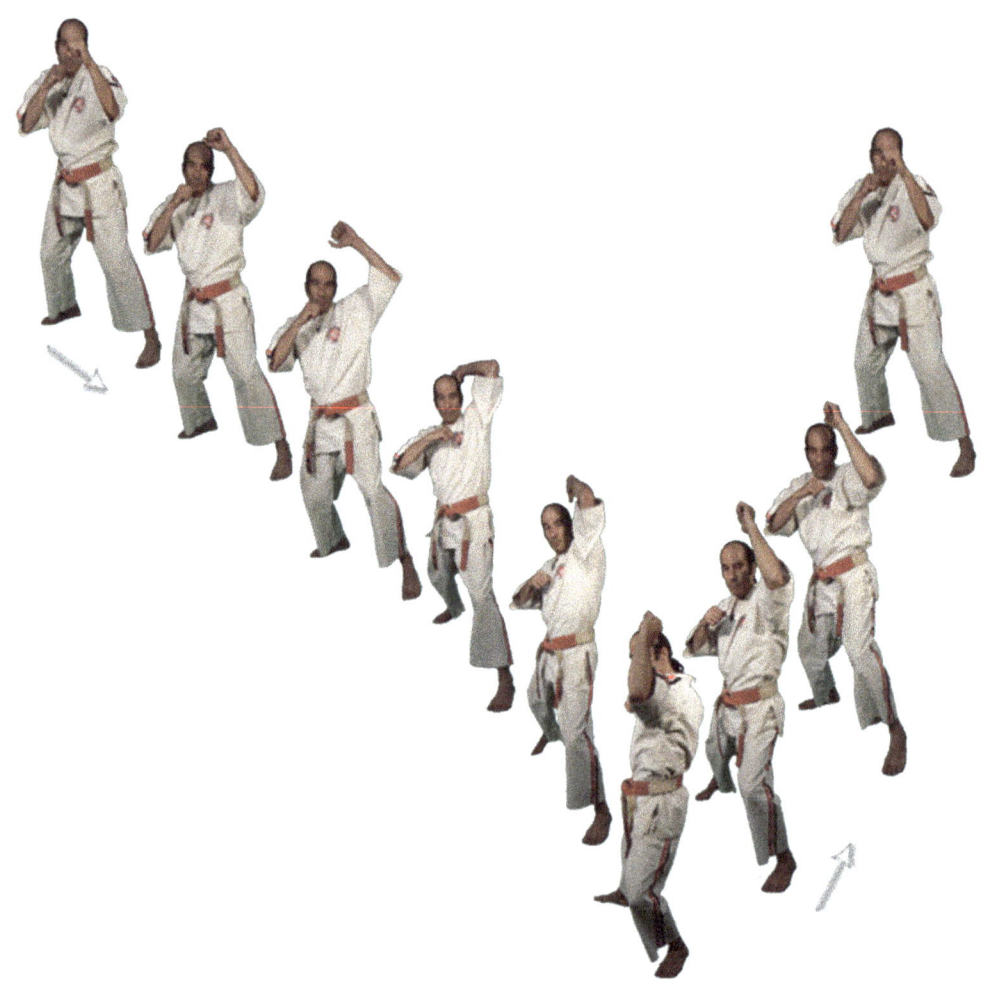

Figure 3.41: Illustrations of the Oi Otoshi Empi Uchi, from the front view.

OI OTOSHI EMPI UCHI: SIDE VIEW

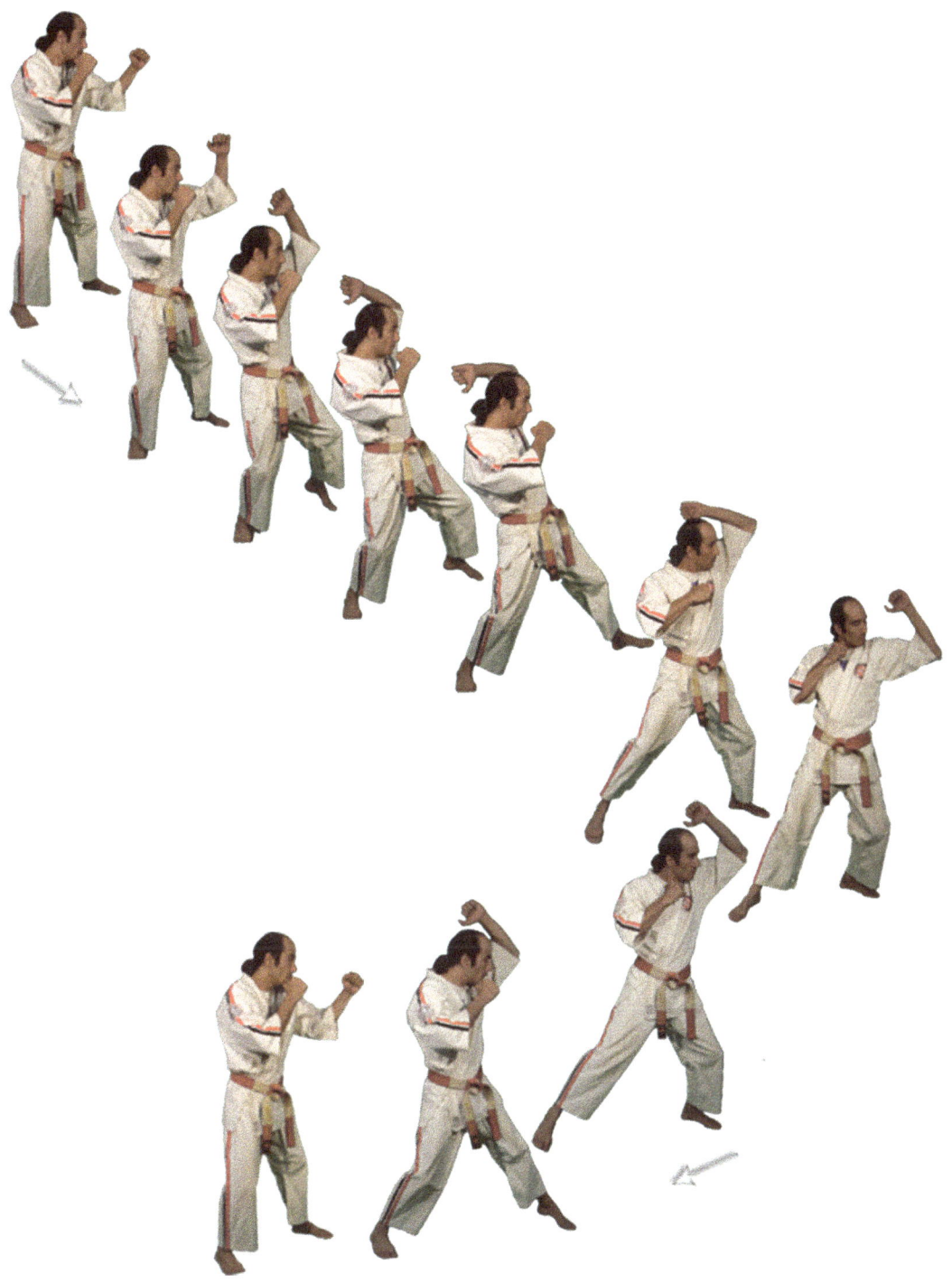

Figure 3.42: Illustrations of the Oi Otoshi Empi Uchi, from the side view.

R. _Hineri Otoshi Empi Uchi (Twist Downward Elbow Strike, Downward Elbow with the Back Hand)_

From a left fighting stance centered to the target, one must push off the right foot stepping forward with the left foot and placing it at the necessary distance from the target keeping it in line (as with all techniques) with the left side of the opponent's body. At the same time, one must lift the right elbow above the height of the target with the palm of the hand above the right ear with the elbow fully bent.

As the left foot lands, one must immediately rotate the hips and shoulders in a counter clockwise direction driving the elbow down onto the target, timing contact when the hips and shoulders are in a straight line with the target. The front hand contact is made with the back of the elbow which is tightened on contact along with the muscles and tendons of the hand and wrist. After making contact, one must retract the technique and step back into a left fighting stance. One must perform all movements in reverse from a right fighting stance for a left twist downward elbow strike. See Figures 3.43 and 3.44 (below) and video for illustration of Hineri Otoshi Empi Uchi.

HINERI OTOSHI EMPI UCHI: FRONT VIEW

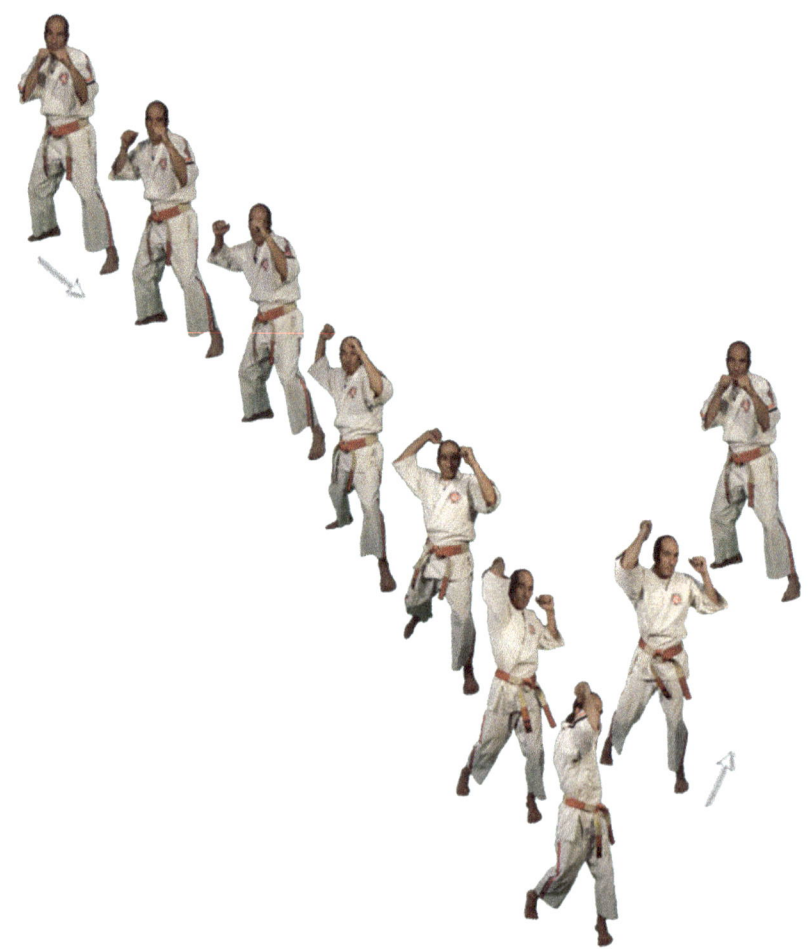

Figure 3.43: Illustrations of the Hineri Otoshi Empi Uchi, from the front view.

HINERI OTOSHI EMPI UCHI: SIDE VIEW

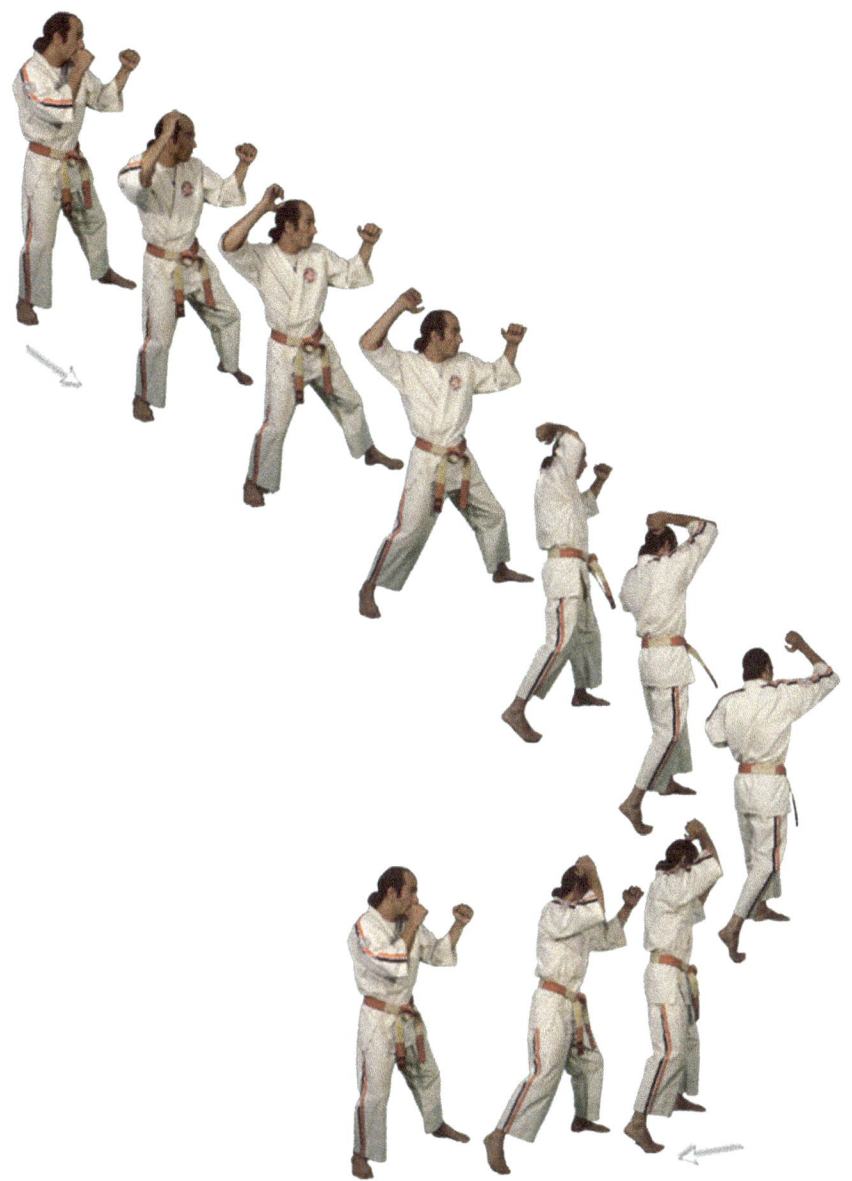

Figure 3.44: Illustrations of the Hineri Otoshi Empi Uchi, from the side view.

S. Hiza Geri (Knee Strikes)

Similar to elbow strikes, knee strikes are very effective close range techniques and are used in most martial arts and fighting competitions. They are mostly used in holding and clinching situations mainly because they can be delivered while holding the opponent with both hands, allowing one to control the opponent's movement when delivering the strike. They are delivered either straight, upward, or circular to the target and like other techniques are driven with the hips and shoulders.

T. Oi Mae Hiza Geri (Lunge Front Knee Strike, Straight Knee Strike with the Front Foot)

From a left fighting stance centered to the target, one must bring the right foot forward and place it close to the left foot making sure that the toes are facing away from the target at approximately 45 degrees and slightly bending the knees so as to lower the center of gravity. The size of this step may vary depending on how far one is from the target. At the same time, one must extend both hands forward and grab the opponent, preferably around the neck layering one hand over the other behind the head and bringing both elbows close together bent at about a 90 degrees angle.

Other grabbing methods can be used such as one hand behind the head and the other either wrapped over or under the opponent's arm, however the two hands clinch behind the head is very effecting for manipulating the opponent's balance and position. Next, one must begin lifting the left knee up towards the target, as the knee is lifted thrust the hips forward as the knee is about to reach the target driving it forward and into the target, at the same time pull the hands in towards the left armpit pulling the opponent's head as the strike makes contact. The shoulders must be slightly pulled back helping balance and allowing the hips to extend further forward. After contact is made, one must quickly put the left foot back to the ground and step back with the right foot into a left fighting stance. Note that this technique can be delivered upward in the same way to a target horizontal to the ground such as pulling the head downwards and striking with the knee in an upwards manner. Perform all movements in reverse from a right fighting stance for a right lunge front knee strike. See Figures 3.45 and 3.46 (below) and video for illustration of Oi Hiza Geri.

OI MAE HIZA GERI: FRONT VIEW

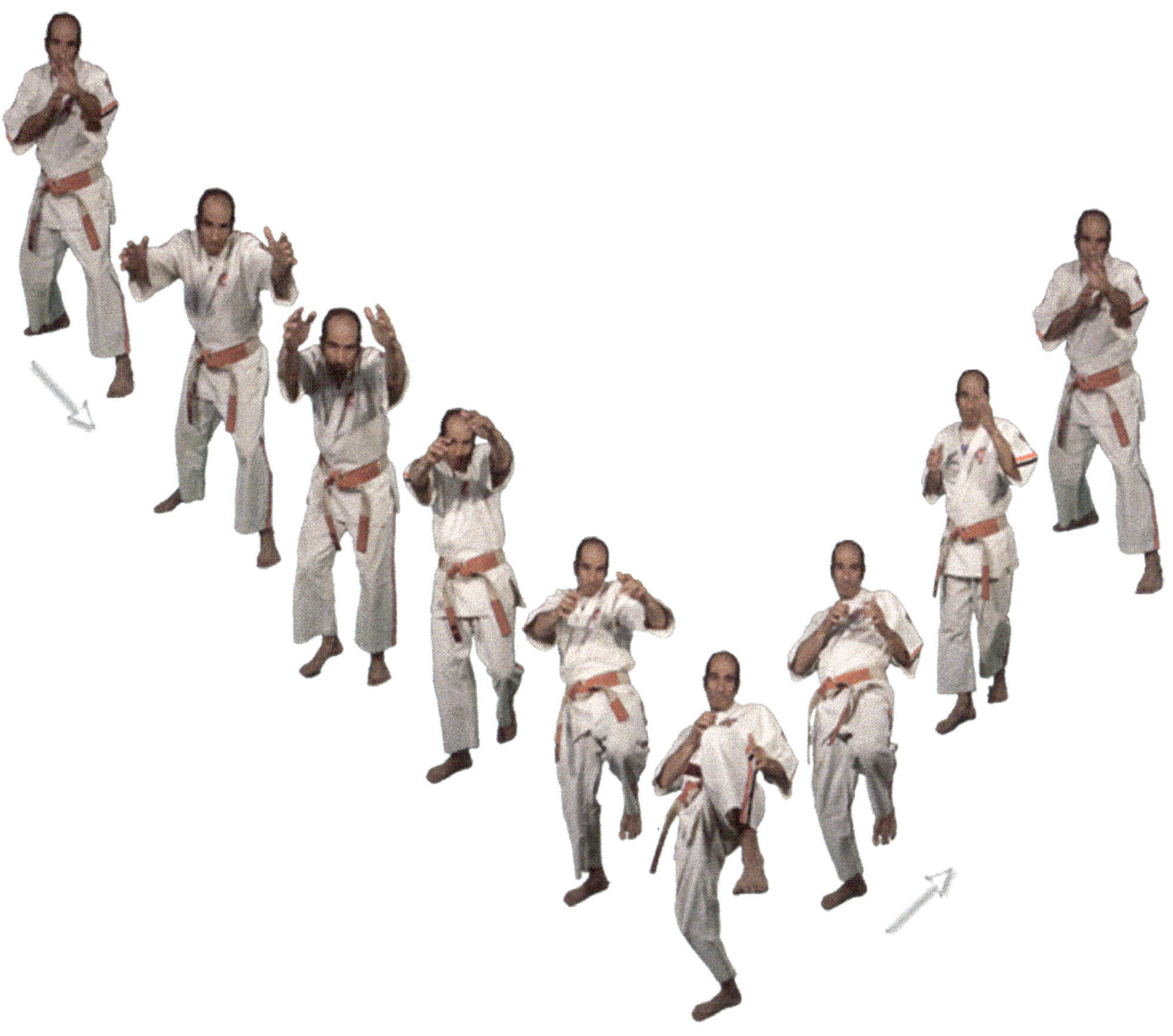

Figure 3.45: Illustrations of the Oi Mae Hiza Geri, from the front view.

OI MAE HIZA GERI: SIDE VIEW

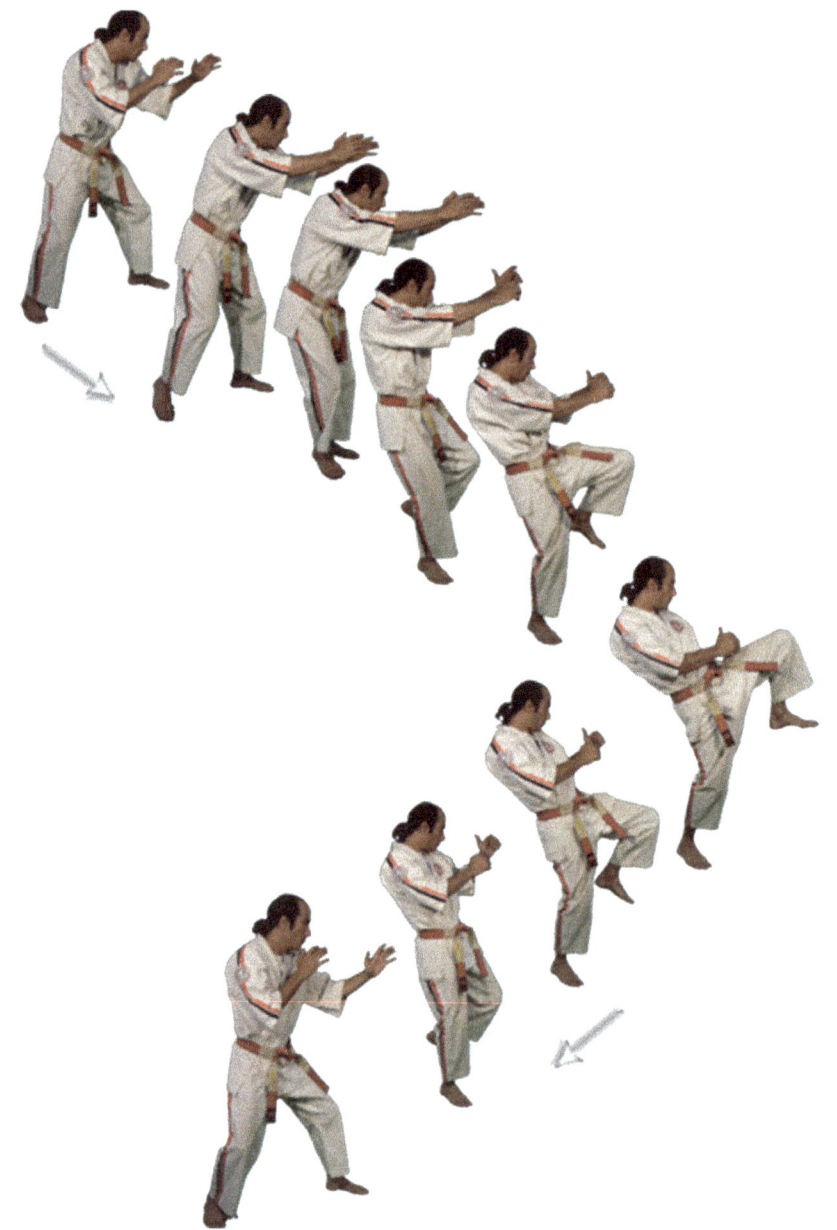

Figure 3.46: Illustrations of the Oi Mae Hiza Geri, from the side view.

U. Hineri Mae Hiza Geri (Twist Front Knee Strike, Straight Knee with the Back Foot)

From a left fighting stance centered to the target, one must push off the right foot, stepping forward with the left foot in line with the left side of the opponent's body, placing it at the necessary distance from the target with the toes pointing 45 degrees away from the target and slightly bend the knees so as to lower the center of gravity. At the same time, one must extend both hands forward and grab the opponent, preferably around the neck layering one hand over the other behind the head and bringing both elbows close together bent at about a 90 degrees angle. Next, one must begin lifting the right knee up towards the target, as the knee is lifted thrust the hips forward as the knee is about to reach the target driving it forward and into the target, at the same time pull the hands in towards the right armpit pulling the opponents head as the strike makes contact. The shoulders are slightly pulled back helping balance and allowing the hips to extend further forward. After contact is made, one must quickly put the right foot back to the ground into a left fighting stance. As with the front leg it can be delivered in an upward manner for a horizontal target. Perform all movements in reverse from a right fighting stance for a left twist front knee strike. See Figures 3.47 and 3.48 (below) and video for illustrations of Hineri Mae Hiza Geri.

HINERI MAE HIZA GERI: FRONT VIEW

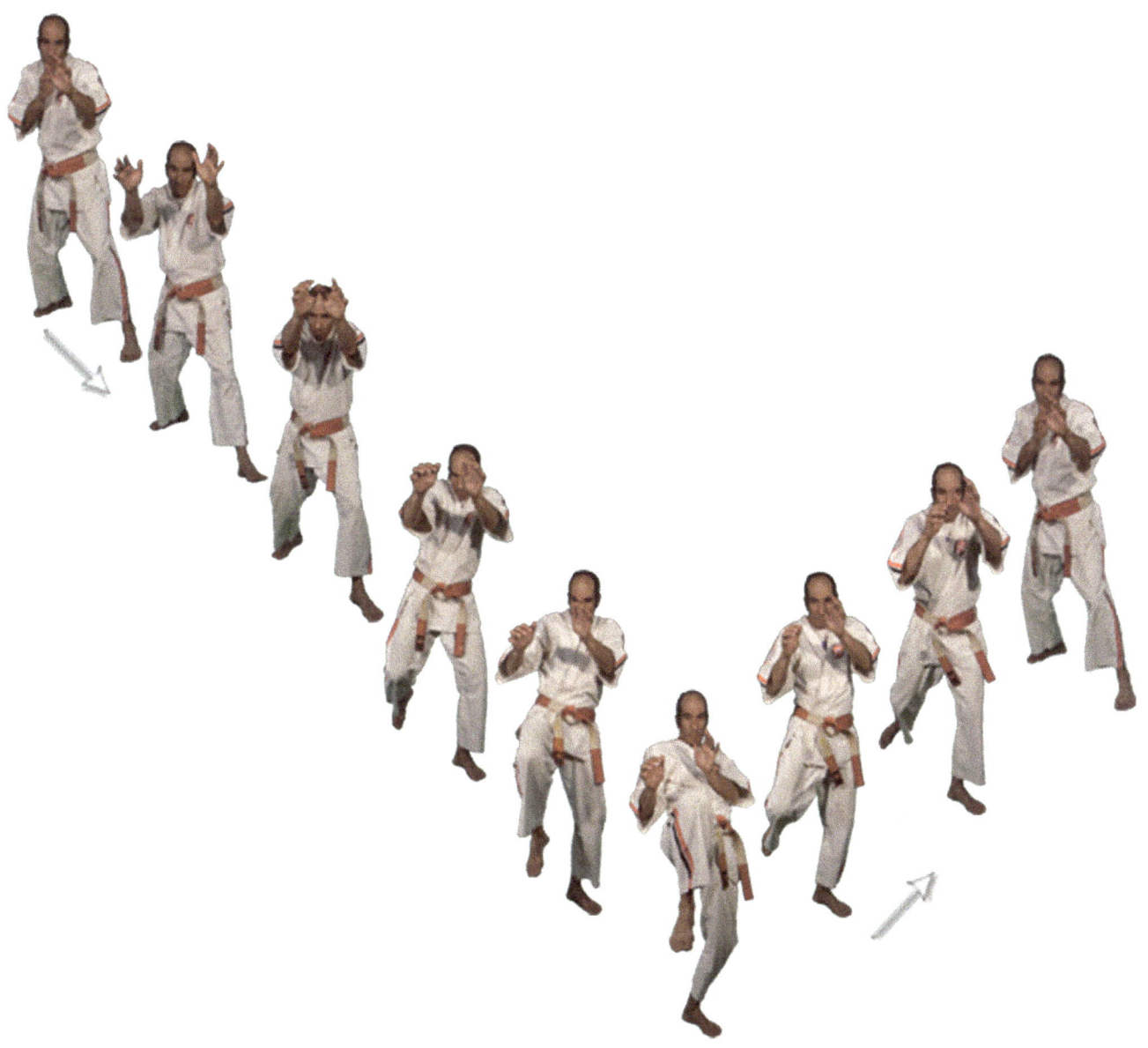

Figure 3.47: Illustrations of Hineri Mae Hiza Geri, from the front view.

HINERI MAE HIZA GERI: SIDE VIEW

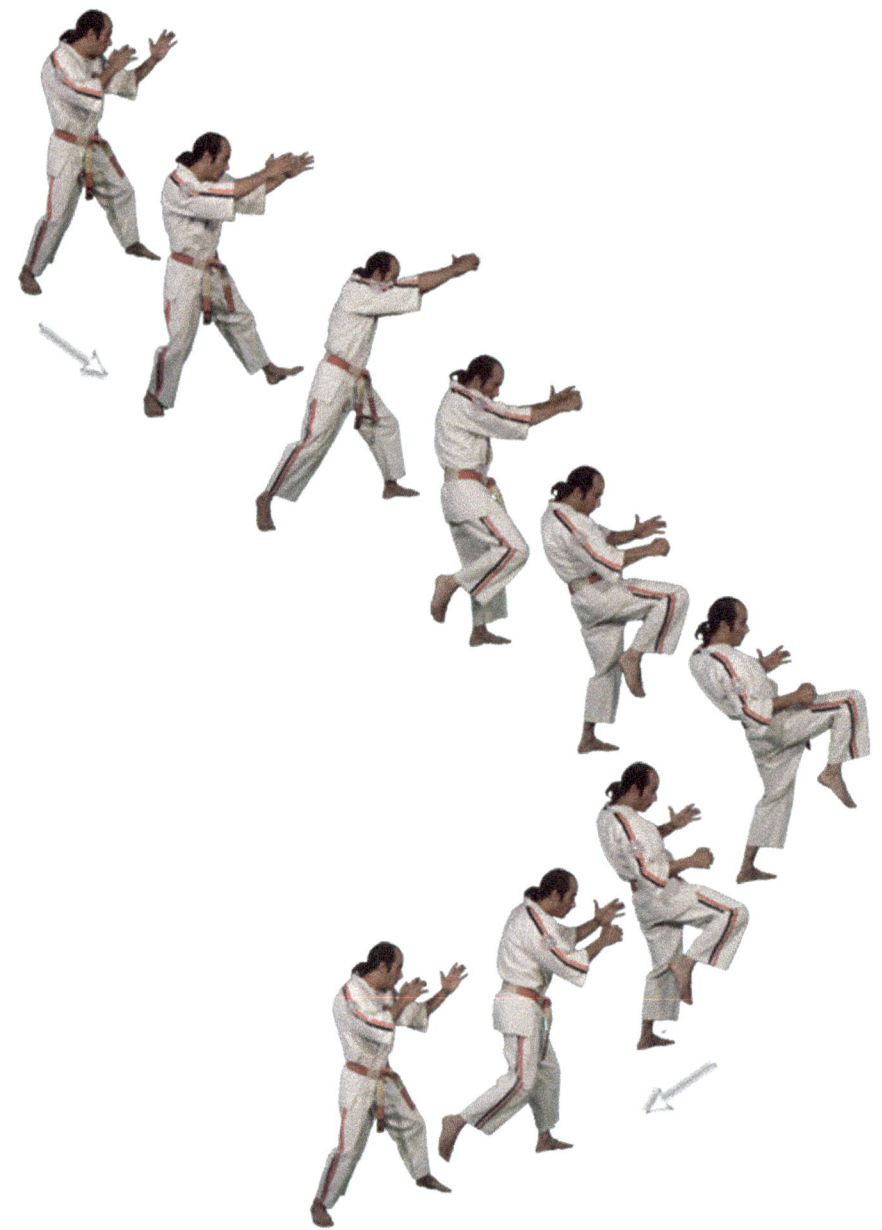

Figure 3.48: Illustrations of Hineri Mae Hiza Geri, from the side view.

V. *Mawashi Hiza Geri (Roundhouse Knee Strike)*

The roundhouse knee strike shares very similar mechanics to the roundhouse kick and is used in clinching/grappling situations to deliver the knee strike in a circular motion mainly to the side of the body and rib cage. Like the roundhouse kick, it is best used from and angle to the target. In other words, they are best delivered after stepping off the target line. Stepping left if a fighter is striking with their right knee and stepping right when striking with the left knee. As with the roundhouse kick the supporting foot should be rotated to allow the weight of the body to be delivered with the strike.

W. Hineri Mawashi Hiza Geri (Twist Roundhouse Knee Strike, Roundhouse Knee with the Back Leg)

From a left fighting stance centered to the target, one must push off the right leg stepping forward and slightly left of the target with the left foot toes pointing slightly left of the target, placing it at the correct distance from the target to deliver the knee strike with the right leg. At the same time extend both hands forward and grab the opponent, preferably around the neck layering one hand over the other behind the head and bringing both elbows close together bent at about a 90 degrees angle and shift the opponent's head towards the right armpit. Next begin lifting up the right knee slightly to the right of the target, as the knee is lifted immediately pivot the left foot and rotate the hips in a counter clockwise direction driving the knee in a circular motion into the target. After contact is made place the right foot back to the ground in a left fighting stance. Perform all movements in reverse from a right fighting stance for a left twist roundhouse knee strike. See Figures 3.49 and 3.50 (below) and video for illustration of Hineri Mawashi Hiza Geri.

HINERI MAWASHI HIZA GERI: FRONT VIEW

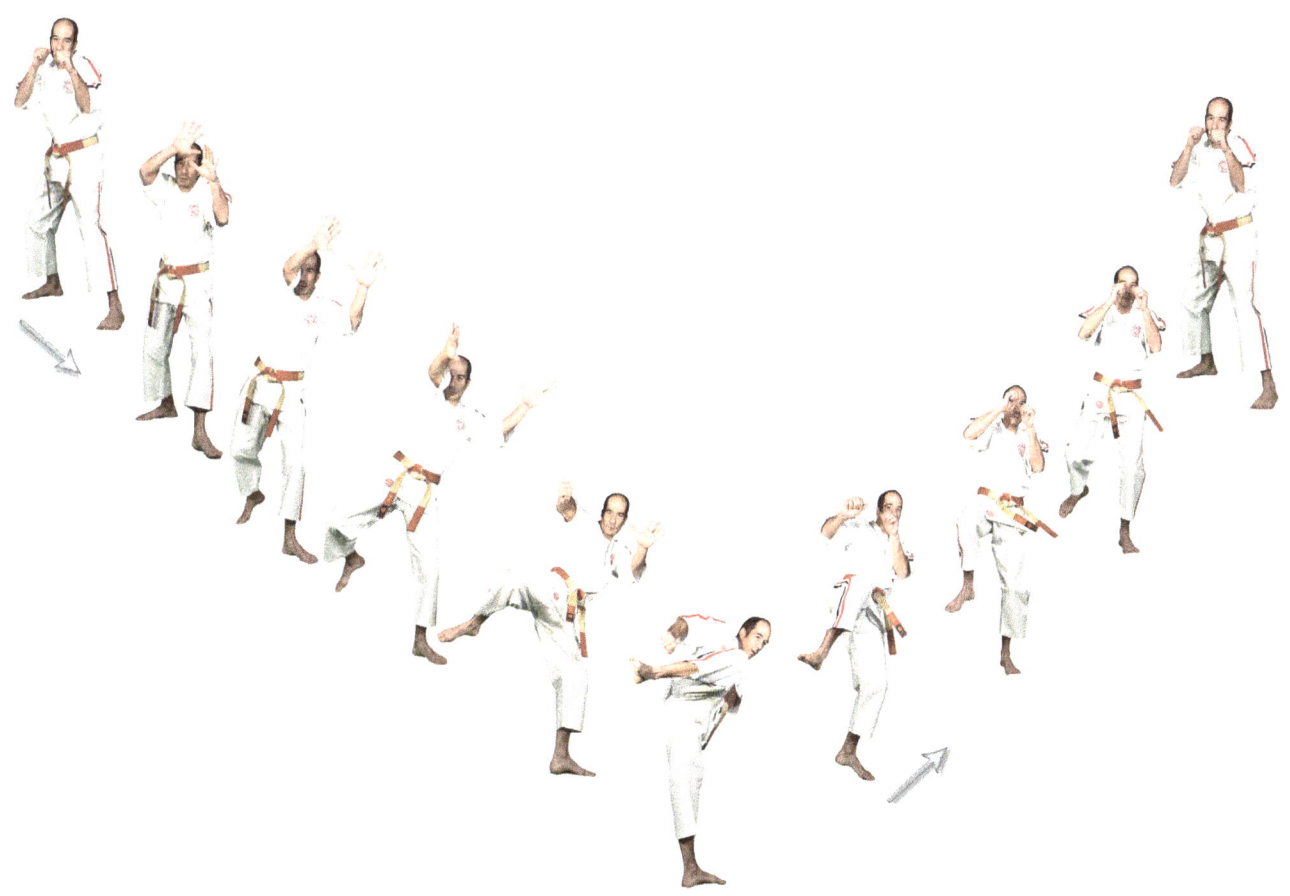

Figure 3.49: Illustrations of Hineri Mawashi Hiza Geri, from the front view.

HINERI MAWASHI HIZA GERI: SIDE VIEW

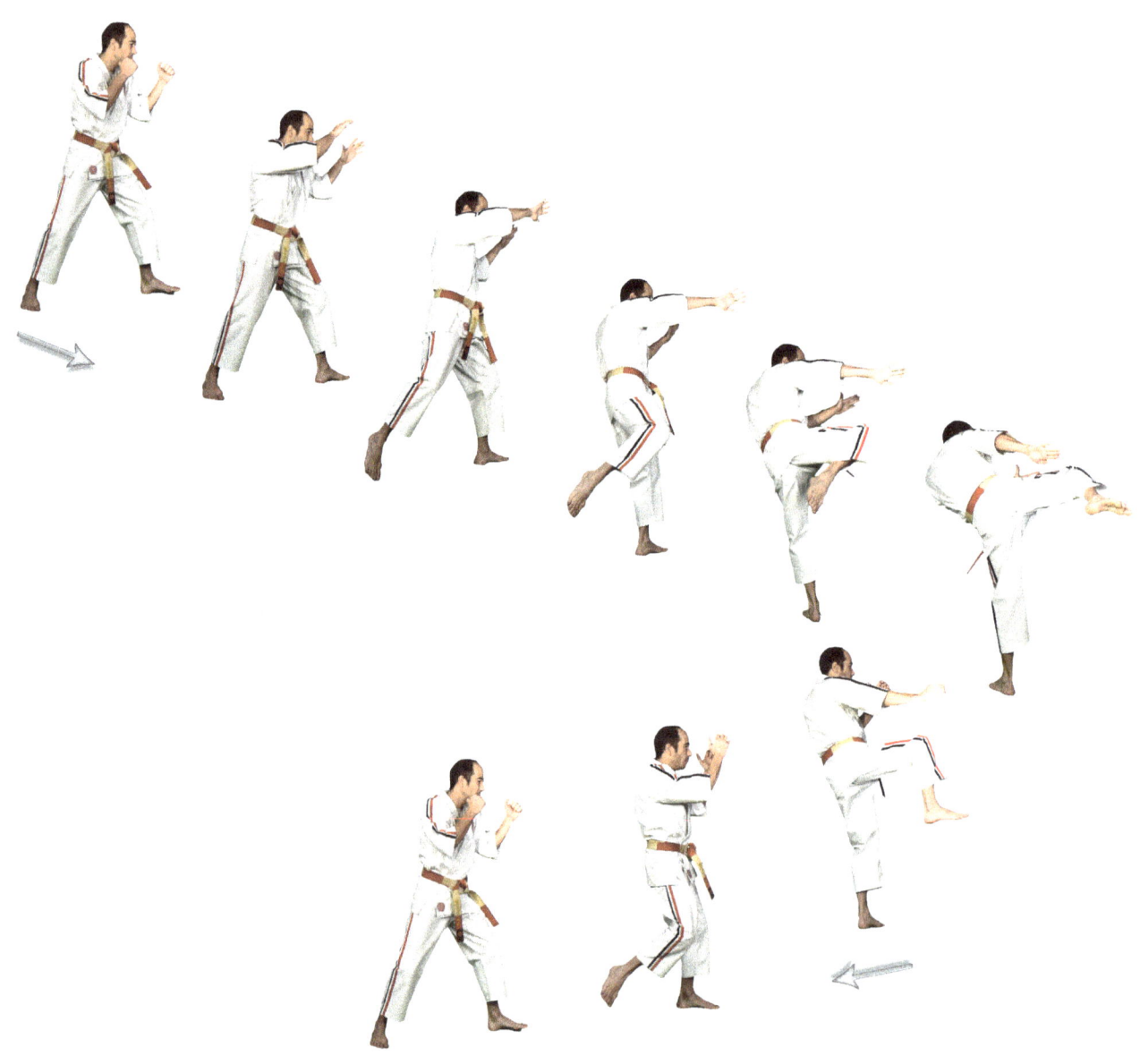

Figure 3.50: Illustrations of Hineri Mawashi Hiza Geri, from the side view.

CHAPTER SUMMARY

Having now examined all the basic punching, kicking, and striking techniques, it should now be understood that all techniques share the same fundamentals in terms of maximizing power by allowing for the use of one's full body weight and maximizing the speed of that technique on contact. All techniques must be built into one fluid motion and an intentional focus must be placed to build the relaxation of the striking limb right up until the moment of contact.

Another important factor is to harmonize one's movement with the delivery of each technique. The techniques in this chapter have all been described from one range to show continuity, however it is important to practice all basic techniques with the different types of foot work covering different distances and harmonizing that footwork with the different techniques. This will help a fighter to identify which techniques are preferable at different distances and how to most effectively cover the distance presented. It is also important to practice all techniques from a close range where no step is required and preferably from a front facing natural stance. This will help to isolate the hip and body movement as there will be no momentum started by the step and will thus force one to develop the power from the hip and body movement. See video for illustration of techniques applied with the different footwork and distances.

Lastly, when training in all basic techniques, it is important to develop the ability to deliver these techniques not only when attacking or moving forward as described in the basic techniques above, but also while moving backwards or in a defensive manner. Again, the footwork used when moving backwards must be harmonized with the techniques and the timing developed for striking while moving forward and backward. See video for illustrations of basic techniques when moving backward.

CHAPTER 4: OFFENSIVE FIGHTING

ONCE THE BASIC techniques are learned, the next step is building a strong foundation for contact fighting and self-defense and developing effective offensive and defensive strategies for practical applications. A fighter must decide the best strategy whether offensive or defensive depending on the attributes possessed by the opponent to maximize their chance of success. First, this chapter will look at offensive fighting and the principles used for successful attacking strategies. While a strong offensive strategy can be very effective, there are certain risks inherent when initiating contact in a fighting situation, the main one being the risk of counterattack. When a fighter initiates an attack, the opponent's reactions can be unpredictable. Oftentimes, it is also easy to be preoccupied by executing one's own attack that one fails to expect or prepare for the counterattack. For instance, a fighter may get hit when moving forward, which can add impact to the strike making it a particularly undesirable time to receive a strong blow. As such, it is important to develop techniques and strategies to minimize these dangers. This can be done first, by using strategies for disrupting an opponent's abilities to strike when entering the striking zone and second, by building sensible combinations of techniques that allow one to follow the opponent's movements, keeping them in a defensive posture and making it difficult for them to find an opening to counter.

4.1 ENTRY TECHNIQUES: TSUKURI, KUZUSHI, KIME (SET-UP, OFF-BALANCE, EXECUTION)

Entry techniques are a key concept that are taught in many Japanese Budo arts and used for many different applications. For instance, it is used in Judo with the off-balance occurring first, followed by the set-up and then, the execution of the technique. The difference is that in Judo, the opponents are already grabbing each other whereas in striking, the distance must be covered before a technique can be executed. As applied to striking, the term Tsukuri means to set-up and it refers to the footwork used to put a fighter in position to strike. Kuzushi means to off-balance or break through the opponent's defense or guards. Finally, Kime means to execute the selected technique. As with similar concepts described earlier in this book, this concept must be developed into a fast fluid motion like a whip or wave.

There are several different techniques used to create kuzushi (i.e. an opening for attack), they consist of either attacking the guard (hands and arms) or attacking the legs, also known as "leg checking". When "leg checking", a variation of the roundhouse kick is used to break the opponent's balance creating an opening for attack. The main difference with the low roundhouse kick and the "leg check" is that the low kick is driven into the muscle of the keg to create damage to the leg, whereas the "leg check" is used to the lower part of the calf muscle to bump the leg in the direction of the toes to momentarily throw an opponent off balance.

4.1.1 HAND KUZUSHI (OFF-BALANCING BY ATTACKING THE ARMS OR GUARD)

These types of entry techniques are very useful against opponents with strong guard positions where their hands are somewhat outstretched from their bodies. This is typical when a fighter is trying to maintain distance while blocking or deflecting one's attack. In this way, the guarding hand is knocked down with the non-striking hand, just prior to the execution of the technique, rendering that hand unable to block or cover the target. See Figure 4.1 for details.

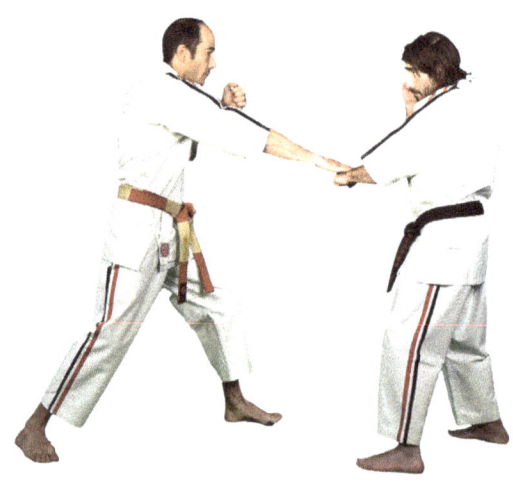

Figure 4.1: Hand Kuzushi showing Off-balancing by attacking the arms or guard.

4.1.2 KUZUSHI WITH THE FRONT HAND

When executing kuzushi with the front hand, the most effective techniques that can be used to follow it are the Twist Front Punch (Hineri Mae Tsuki), the Front leg straight kick (Oi Mae Geri), and the Twist Roundhouse kick (Hineri Mawashi Geri). The choice of which one would depend on the opponent's stance, movement, and reactions. See Figure 4.2 for detailed illustrations.

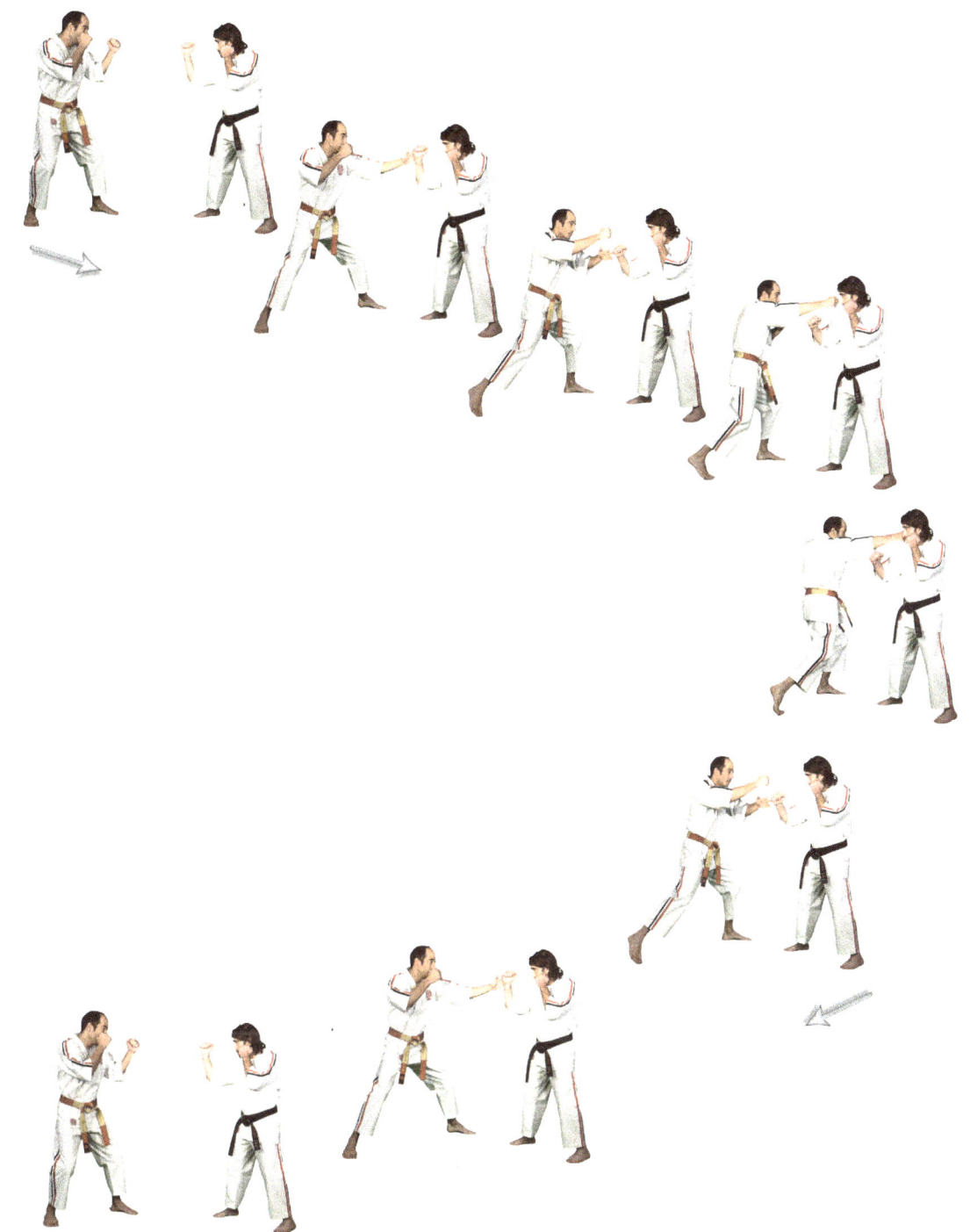

Figure 4.2: Illustrating Kuzushi with the Front Hand

4.1.3 KUZUSHI FROM OPPOSITE STANCE TO THE OPPONENT (EG. LEFT STANCE TO RIGHT STANCE)

From left fighting stance, begin stepping into the striking range using the appropriate step to cover the distance, stepping slightly left of the target. As soon as one's guard hand (left hand) can reach the opponent. Use the palm of the hand to knock the opponent's front hand down and slightly right while still in motion to the target and immediately execute a Right Twist Punch as with the above technique. Entry from the opposite stance favours the Twist Straight Punch and Twist Roundhouse Kick. See Figure 4.1 and the accompanying video for illustration of Hand Kuzushi with the lead hand from the opposite stance and variations of this technique. See Figure 4.3 for detailed illustrations.

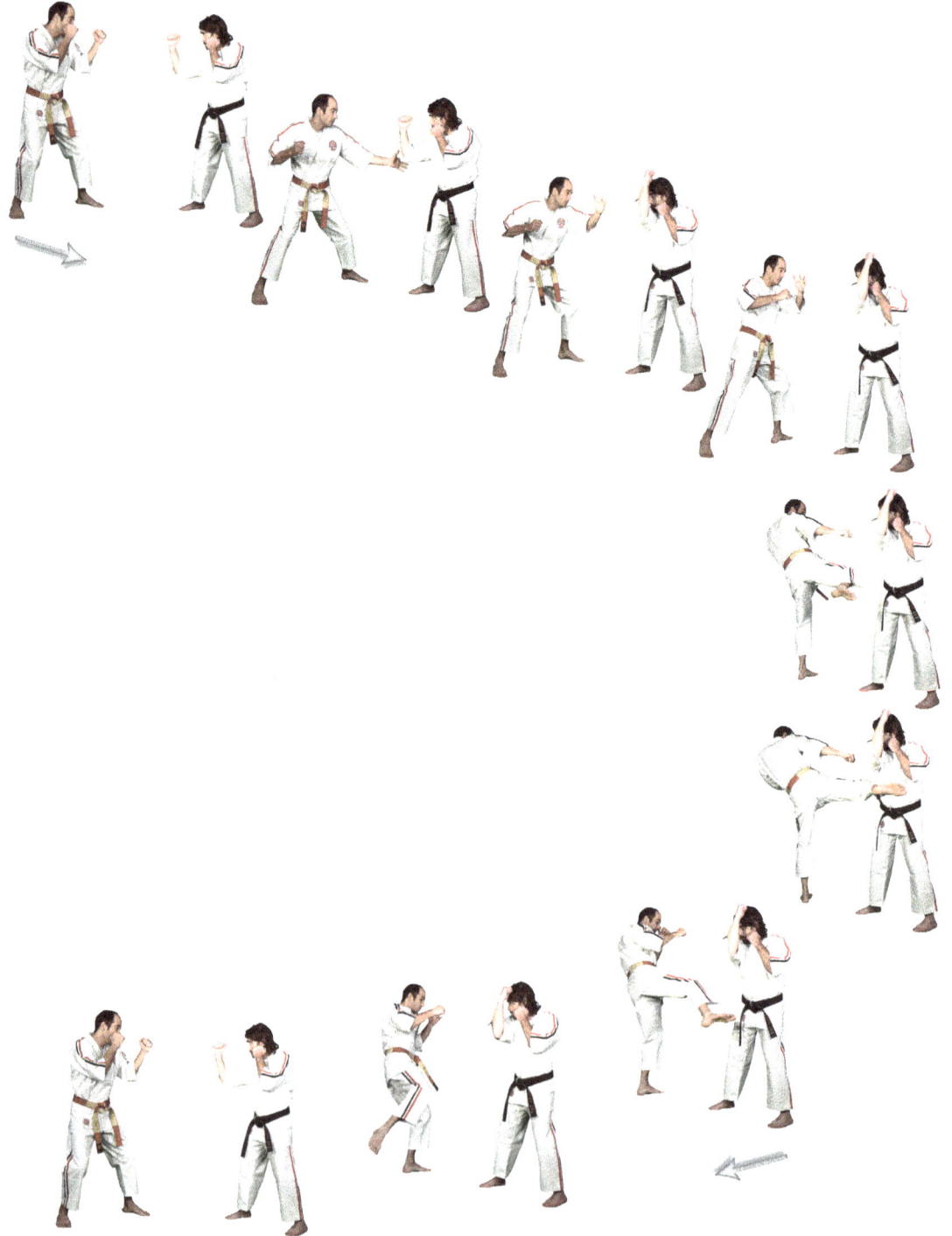

Figure 4.3: Illustrating Front hand Kuzushi from opposite stance with kick attack

4.1.4 KUZUSHI WITH THE BACK HAND

When executing kuzushi with the back hand, the most effective techniques that can be used to follow it are the Lunge Front Punch (Oi Mae Tsuki), the Back Leg Straight Kick (Hineri Mae Geri) and Lunge Roundhouse Kick (Oi Mawashi Geri). The choice of which would depend on the opponent's stance, movement, and reactions.

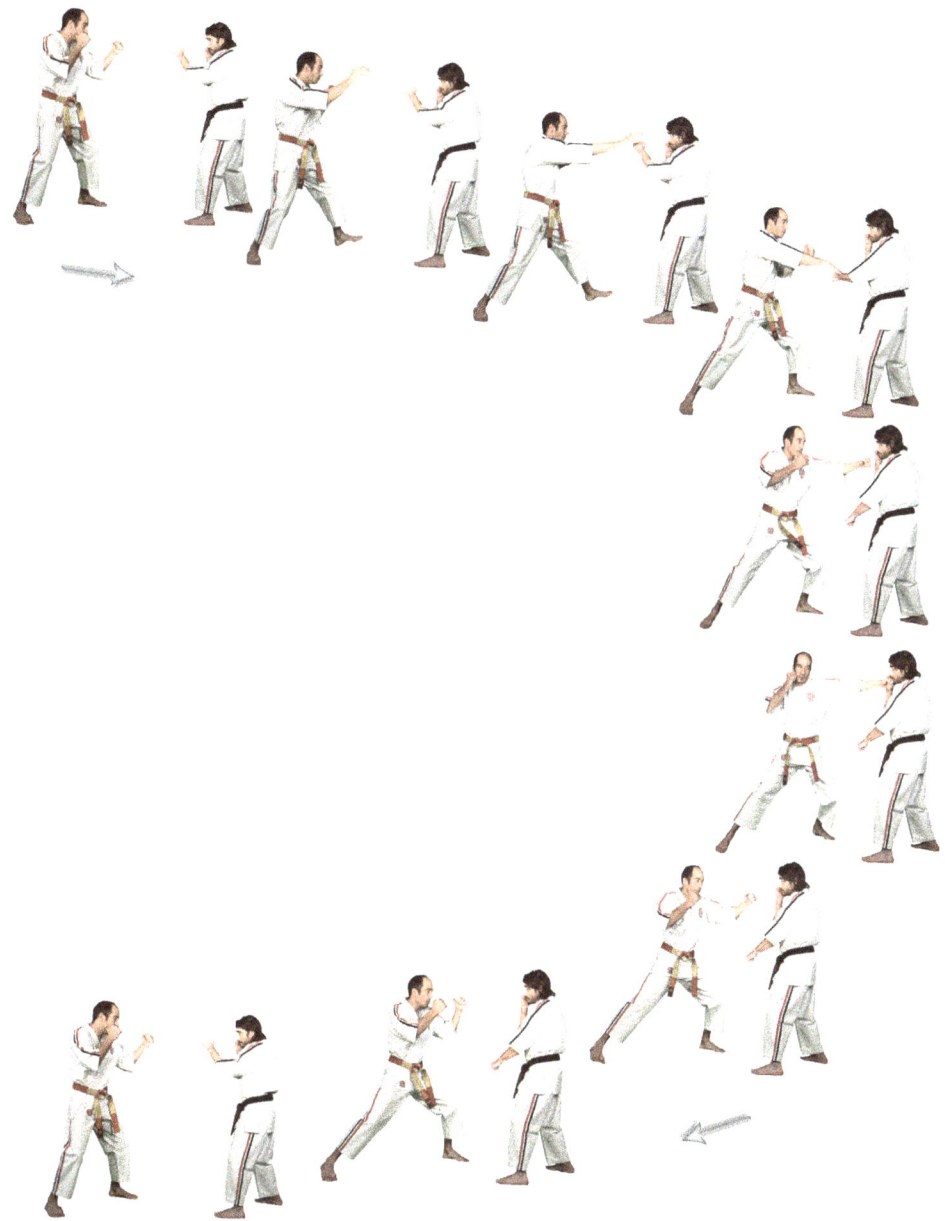

Figure 4.4: Illustrating kuzushi with the back hand.

From Left fighting stance, one must begin by stepping into the striking range while using the appropriate step to cover the distance stepping slightly right of the target. Then, proceed with twisting the hips slightly and rotating the shoulders in a counter clockwise direction. This must be immediately followed by reaching out with the back hand (right hand) and using the palm of the hand to knock the opponent's front hand down and slightly left, while still in motion towards the target, bringing the left hand back to cover the left side of the face. Finally, execute a Left Lunge Straight Punch or one of the above-mentioned techniques for effective use with a back hand kuzushi.

The contact with the opponent's front arm should be made around halfway down the forearm and in a quick hitting motion rather than a pushing motion. This way, the hand can be kept up after knocking down the opponent's guard. The execution of the technique should be timed so that it just passes over the right hand immediately after it knocks down the opponent's hand. See Figure 4.4 and the accompanying video for a detailed illustration of Hand Kuzushi with the back hand and variations with different techniques.

Here is an example of the same Kuzushi, followed by a left roundhouse kick to a body target. It should be noted that targets for techniques can be changed and adjusted to suit the opponent and the situation. In this example, the kick can be delivered to a head target or a leg target in the case of either a shorter or taller opponent. See Figure 4.5.

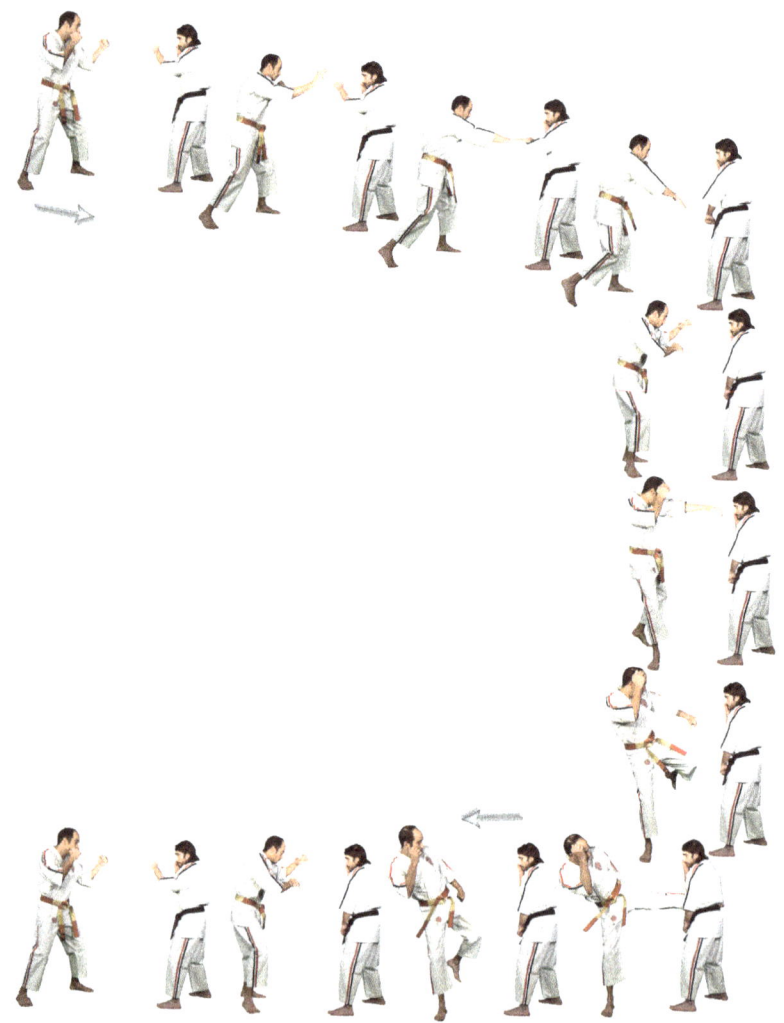

Figure 4.5: Illustrated kuzushi with back hand followed by left roundhouse kick.

4.2 LEG KUZUSHI (OFF-BALANCING BY ATTACKING THE LEGS, "LEG-CHECKS")

The primary concept of leg-checking involves throwing one's opponent off-balance momentarily just as one is attacking, by using a quick snapping roundhouse kick to shift the opponent's front leg in a direction that disrupts their center of gravity. The striking technique can then be immediately executed while the opponent is trying to regain balance. It can be done either to the inside or the outside of the opponent's front leg and can be followed up by a straight punch or roundhouse kick. As opposed to the roundhouse kick, during leg-checking, contact is made with the lower part of the opponent's leg, about halfway up the calf muscle and must be delivered in the direction in which the opponent's toes are facing or as close to that direction as possible. It is helpful to use one's curve of the ankle and foot when making contact for the leg-check because it will create a kind of hooking effect allowing one to hit the leg easier in the direction of the toes which is somewhat back in one's own direction and to the side. It is important to pull back the kicking foot as quickly as possible regaining a centered and balanced stance so that the chosen technique can be executed as quickly as possible, before the opponent regains balance. For this purpose, leg checks are not thrown with full power but as mentioned above with a quick snapping motion which allows quicker recovery. See Figure 4.6 for illustrations.

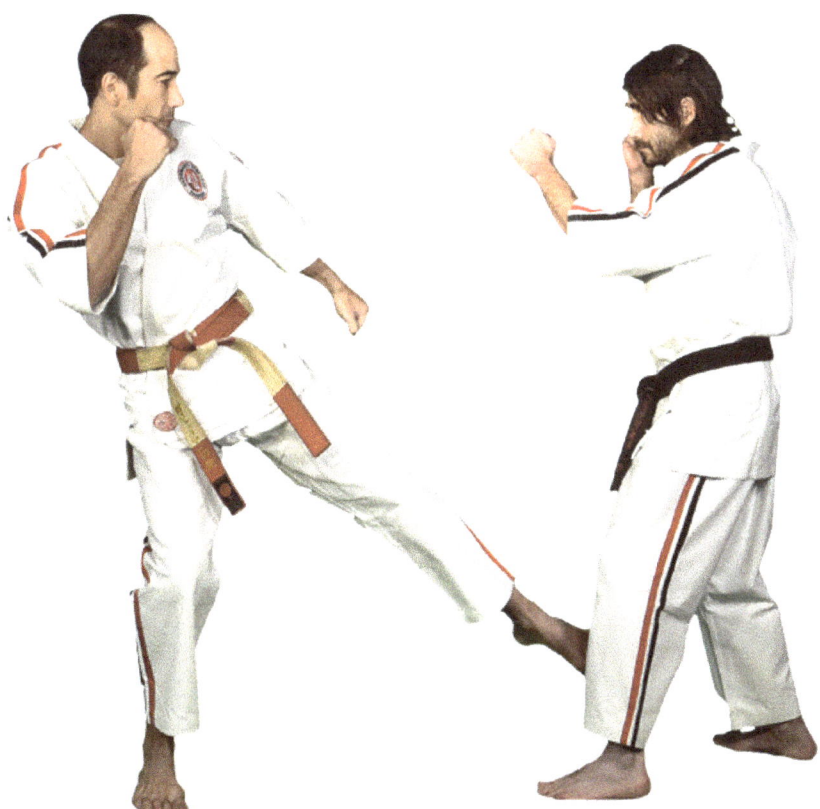

Figure 4.6: Illustration of Leg Kuzushi.

4.2.1 INSIDE LEG CHECKS

From a left fighting stance centered to the target, one must bring the right foot forward as far as necessary to put one in kicking distance of the opponent's front leg. Note that this distance will be closer than a body target and therefore requires a smaller step. Immediately execute the left roundhouse kick keeping the foot close to the ground and strike the inside of the calf muscle hitting the leg to the right and slightly back towards themselves using the crook for the foot and ankle. After making contact, immediately bring the foot back to the left into a balanced left fighting stance and execute either Front or twist straight punch or the twist roundhouse kick. See Figure 4.7 and video for illustration of inside leg check and its variations.

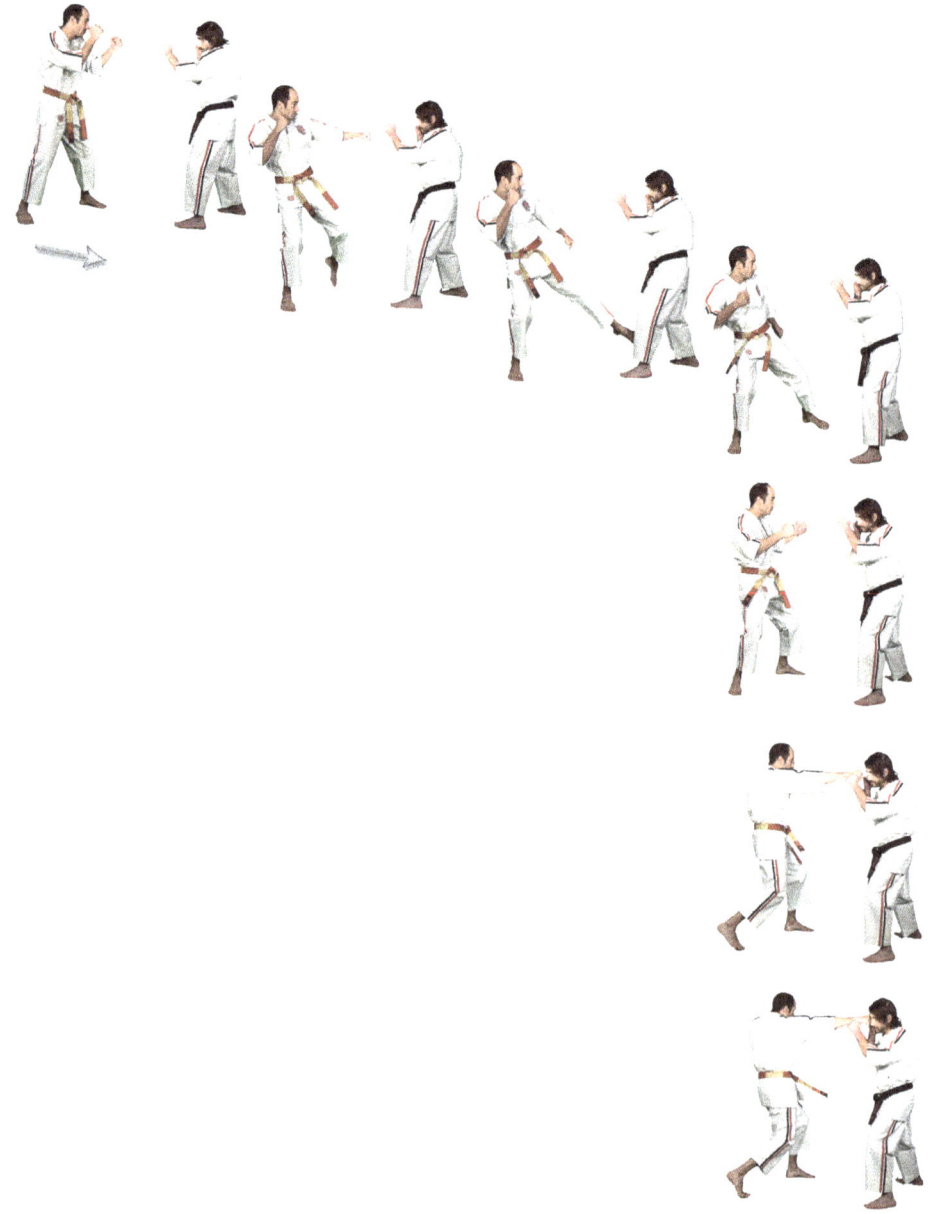

Figure 4.7: Illustration of inside leg check and its variations.

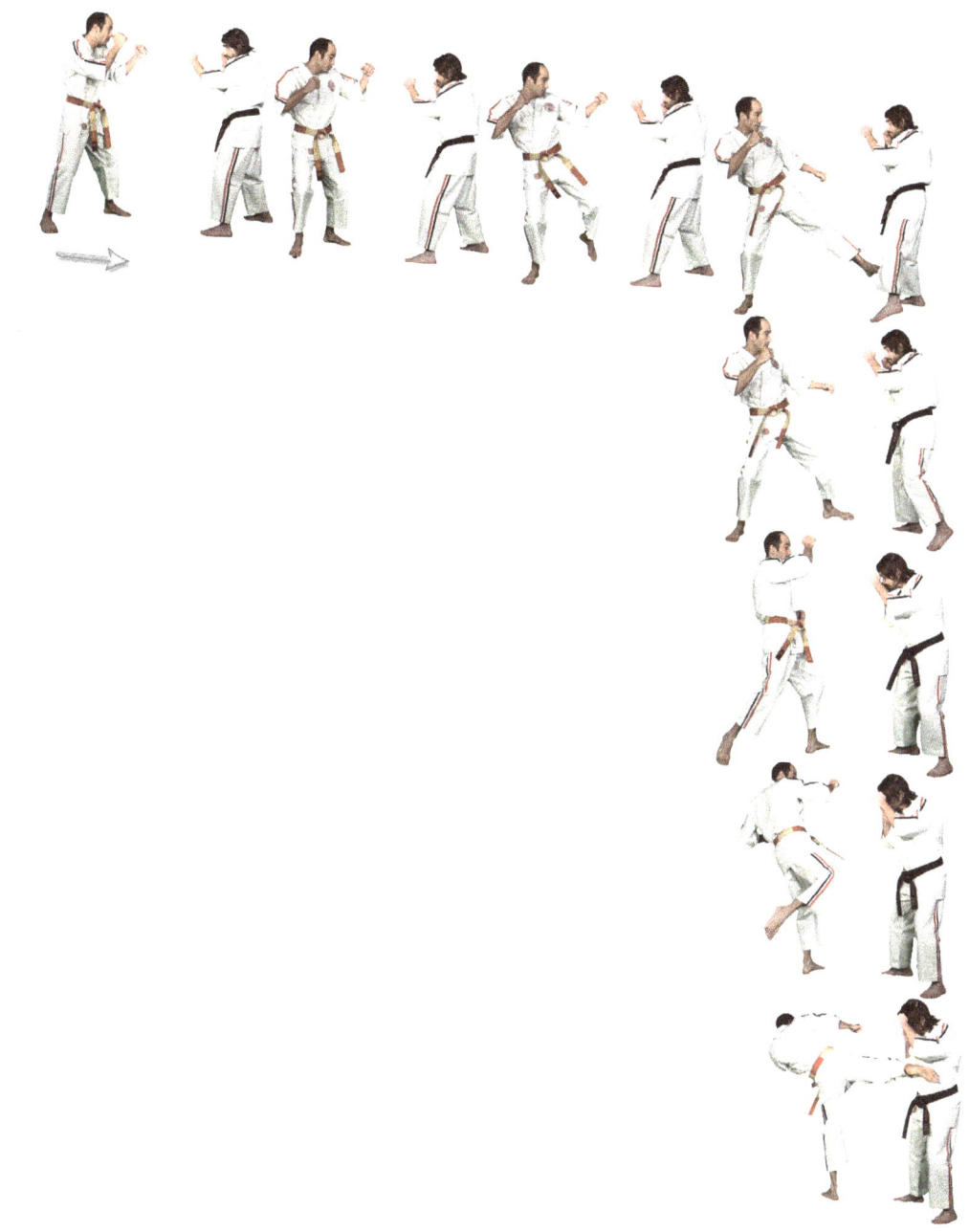

Figure 4.8: Illustration of Inside leg check Kuzushi with kick attack.

4.2.2 OUTSIDE LEG CHECK

From a left fighting stance centered to the target, step with the left foot to adjust the distance and immediately execute a right twist roundhouse kick keeping the foot close to the ground and strike the outside of the calf muscle hitting the leg to the left and slightly back towards themselves using the crook for the foot and ankle. After making contact immediately bring the foot back to the right into a balanced right fighting stance and execute either right Front or left twist straight punch or the left twist roundhouse kick. See Figure 4.9 and video for illustration of outside leg check and its variations.

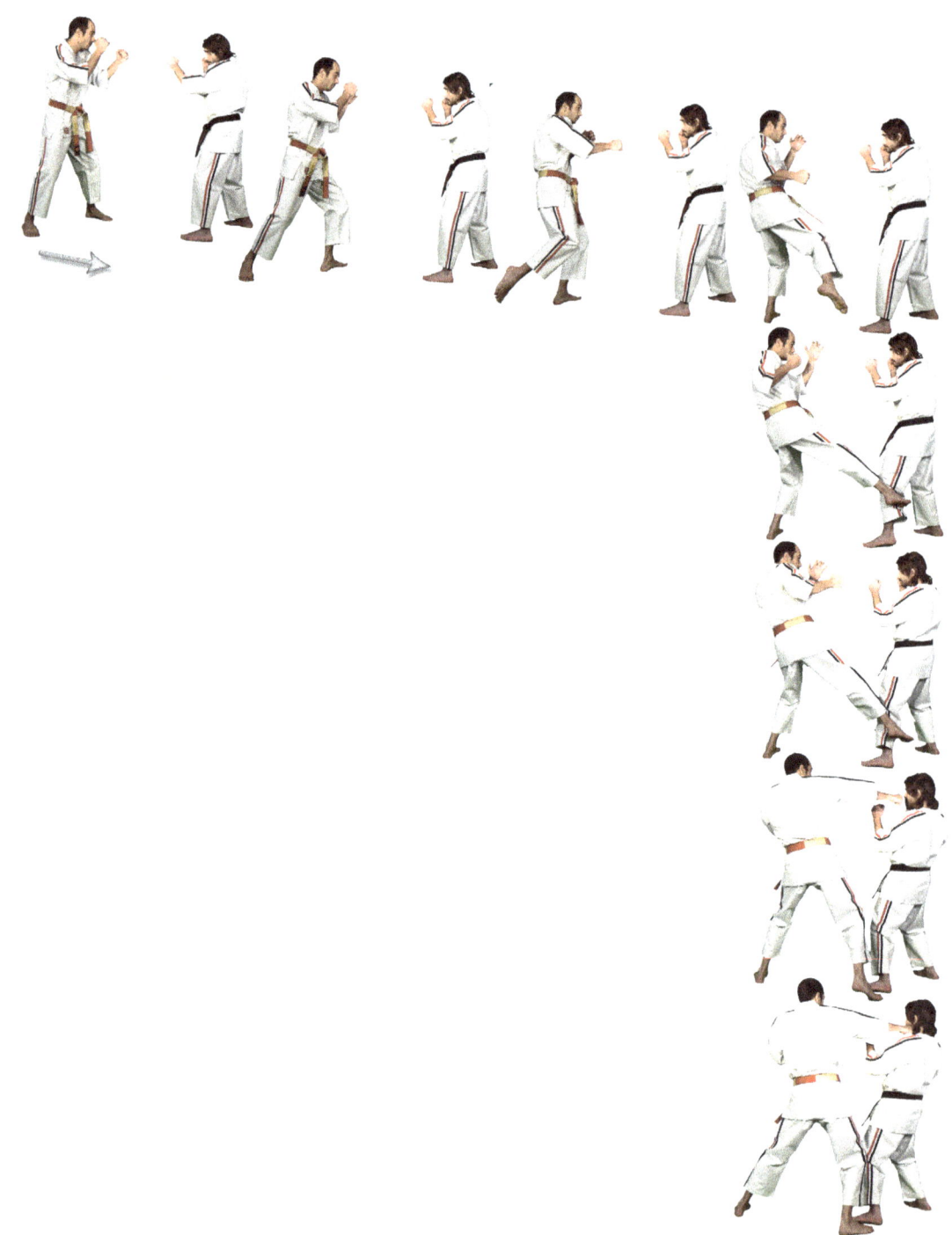

Figure 4.9: Illustration of outside leg check.

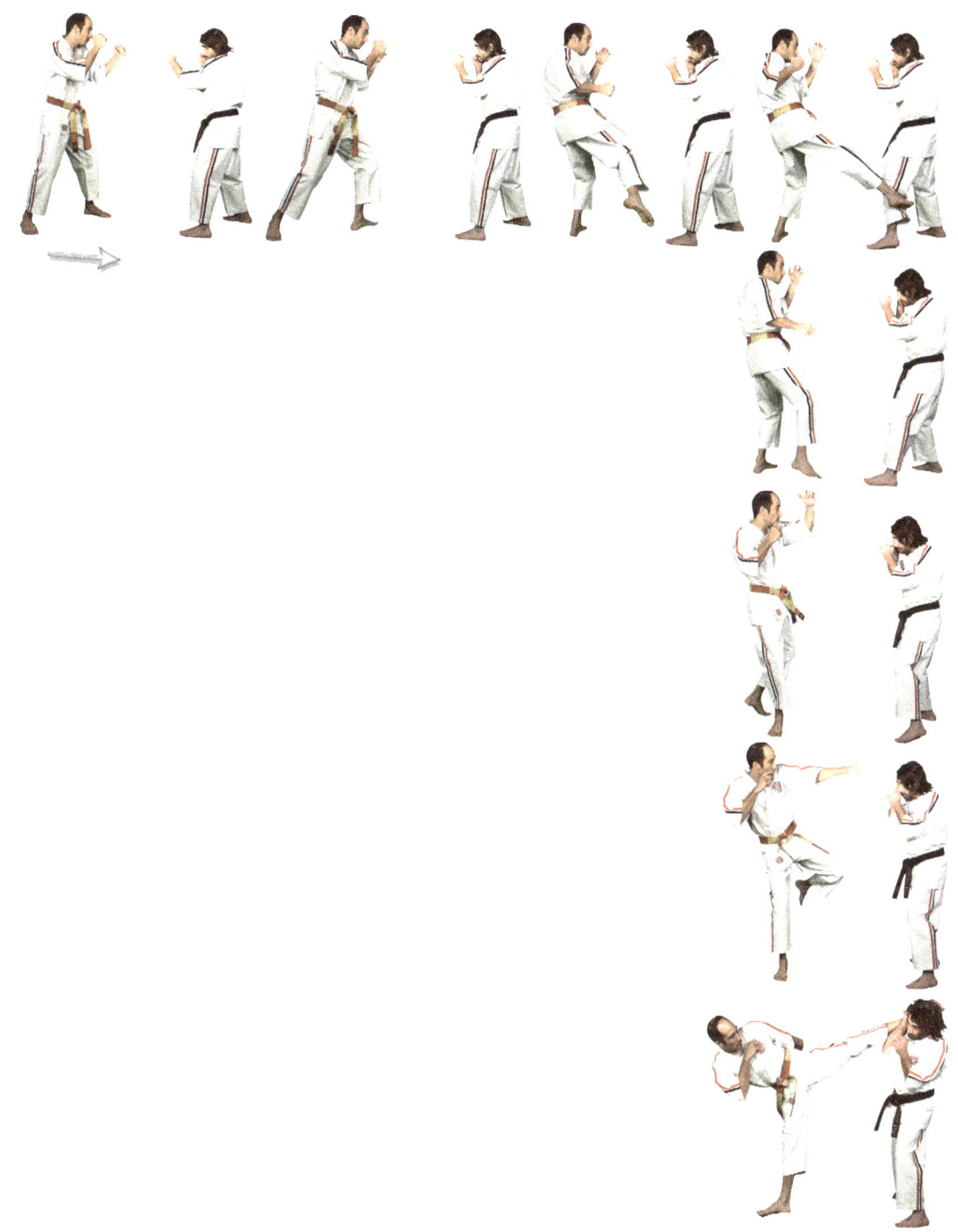

Figure 4.10: Illustration of Outside leg check Kuzushi with kick attack.

4.3 COMBINATIONS

Another important aspect of offensive fighting is the formulation of combinations. By combining speed and momentum generated by entry technique with natural movement of body gives the advantage in overcoming the opponent's movement and defenses. Combinations should utilize different techniques and targets and should have 3 main characteristics. First, the entry technique, second, the scoring or power technique, and third, the finishing or escaping technique. For the purpose of this book, we will look at the most commonly used and effective combination of 2 or 3 techniques. However, by following the basic principles for formulating combinations, one can create combination of as many techniques as needed.

4.4 BASIC PRINCIPLES: HOW TO MAKE COMBINATIONS THAT MAKE SENSE?

The main idea behind formulating combination of techniques is to increase one's chance of landing a perfect technique for attack and minimizing the chance of getting hit in a counterattack. Combination of techniques, therefore, are meant to confuse or trick the opponent so that they are unable to defend themselves from combined techniques. For this purpose, combination of techniques must be smooth and easy transition from one technique to the next. This can be achieved by combining techniques based on the following criteria.

4.4.1 CHANGING TARGETS

An opponent's body has 3 main target levels, Jodan, Chudan and Gidan which simply are, Upper level, middle level, and lower level or Head, Body, and Legs or groin. It is much easier for an opponent to defend multiple techniques that are targeted at the same level. When the target is changed using combined techniques, the opponent must make quick adjustments to their defense, making it harder to avoid multiple techniques in the combination. For this purpose, combination of multiple techniques that changes target throughout each technique e.g. body to head, head to body, head to leg or leg to head etc. is formulated.

4.4.2 CHANGING WEAPONS

As seen in earlier chapters, there are many different weapons used in contact fighting, the fist, foot, knee, elbow etc. It is much easier for an opponent to defend multiple techniques from the same weapon, but by using different weapons one can achieve different distances and overcome the opponent changing the distance in a defensive manner. For this purpose, combinations using different weapons e.g. hand to foot, foot to hand, hand to elbow or knee or other combination of weapons should be used. This will assist in following the opponent's movement and match the distance required.

4.4.3 CHANGING DIRECTION OF ATTACK

As seen in earlier chapters, different techniques are executed in different directions such as straight, round, downward, and upward. It is much easier to defend multiple techniques that comes from the same direction, an opponent can move in a number of directions when attacked. For this reason, combinations that change the direction of attack throughout each technique should be used e.g. straight to round, round to straight, straight to downward or upward etc. This will assist in following the opponent's movement and cutting off their escape.

All 3 of these criteria should be considered when formulating combinations along with change in distance and direction. In this way, the combinations can be tailored to suit the particular strengths and preferences of a specific opponent or based on body size and shape. For example, an opponent who utilizes movement can be cut off by using a straight hand technique to a round foot technique accounting for increase in distance and change in angle. Likewise, an opponent who holds their ground and uses much less movement, can be caught by using a straight or round hand technique, going to a knee or elbow technique which accounts for the short distancing. In short, when formulating combinations by using the principles described above, one will be able to stay in offensive manner while minimizing the opponent's ability to create distance and mount a counterattack.

4.5 BASIC COMBINATIONS

While there are an infinite number of combinations that can be used, it is important to build and develop the basic and most commonly used 2 or 3 techniques combination.

These combinations form the basic foundation for all combinations and teach the body to put together techniques that follow the opponent, cut off escape and maintain favorable distance.

4.6 TWO TECHNIQUES COMBINATION

4.6.1 LEADING WITH THE HANDS

Combo 1: From a left fighting stance, execute a left straight front punch to the head level followed by a right Twist Round House kick to the body level or lower level. When executing the right roundhouse kick, step slightly to the left of the target to create an angle adding power to the kick and getting one off the centerline. This combination works well with an opponent who is stepping to the right. This combo can also be done with the punch to the body and the kick done to the head. See Figure 4.11.

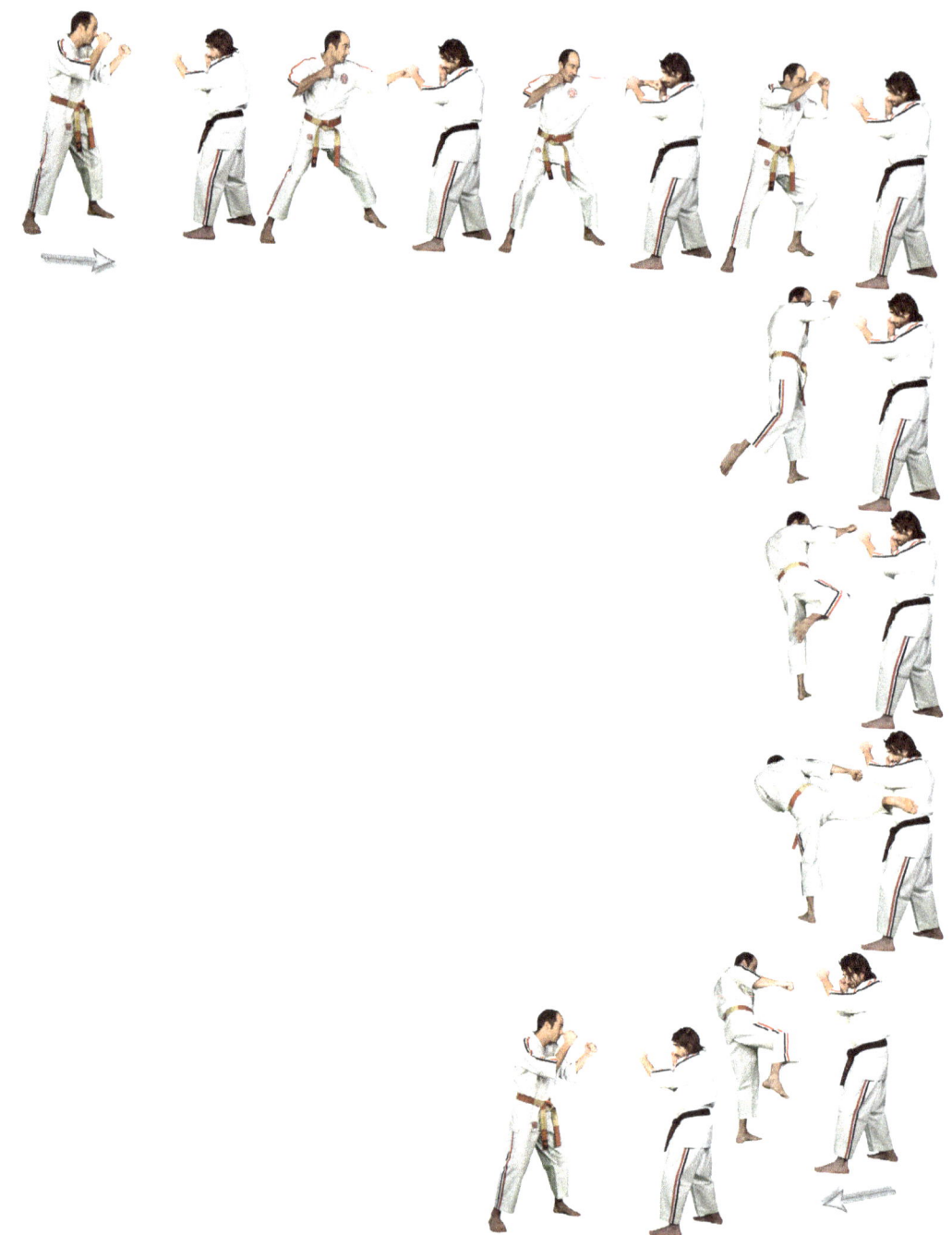

Figure 4.11: Combination of Two Techniques leading with Hands Combo1

Combo 2: From a left fighting stance, execute a right twist straight punch to the head level followed by a left lunge roundhouse kick to the Body level or lower level. As mentioned above, when executing the kick, step slightly to the right of the target to create an angle. This combo also works well with the punch delivered to the body, while dropping the body level throw the kick to the head target. See Figure 4.12.

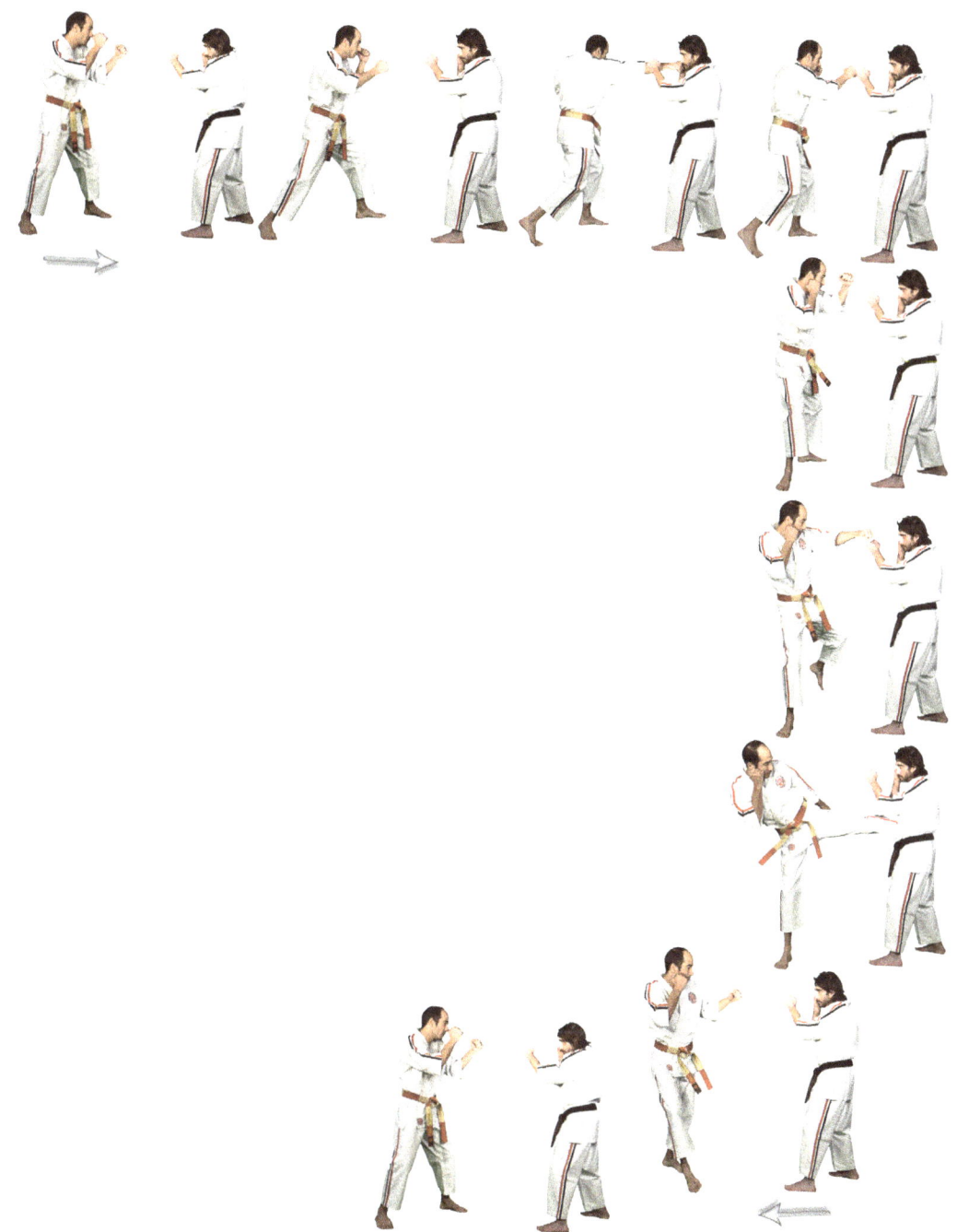

Figure 4.12: Combination of Two Techniques leading with Hands Combo 2

4.6.2 LEADING WITH THE FEET

Combo 3: From a left fighting stance, execute a left lunge roundhouse kick to the body level or lower level. Put the left foot down immediately and execute a right Twist straight punch to the head level. Throw the punch while the kick is still on the way to the ground to minimize the time between the kick and the punch. See Figure 4.13.

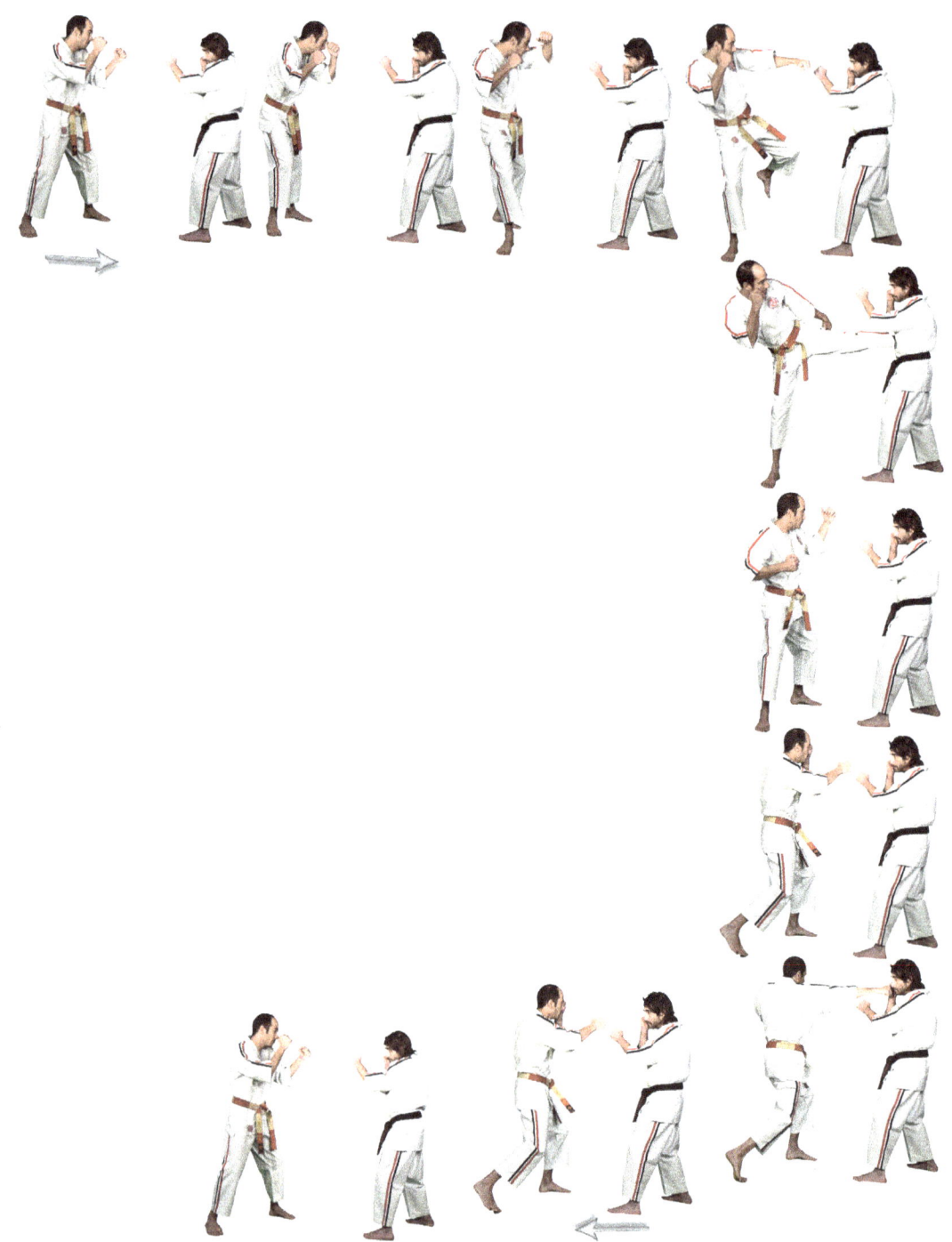

Figure 4.13: Combination of Two Techniques leading with Feet Combo 3

Combo 4: From a left fighting stance, execute a right twist roundhouse kick to the body level or lower level. Put the right foot down immediately in a right fighting stance and execute a left Twist straight punch to the head level. Throwing the punch while the kick is still on the way to the ground will minimize the time between the kick and the punch. See Figure 4.14.

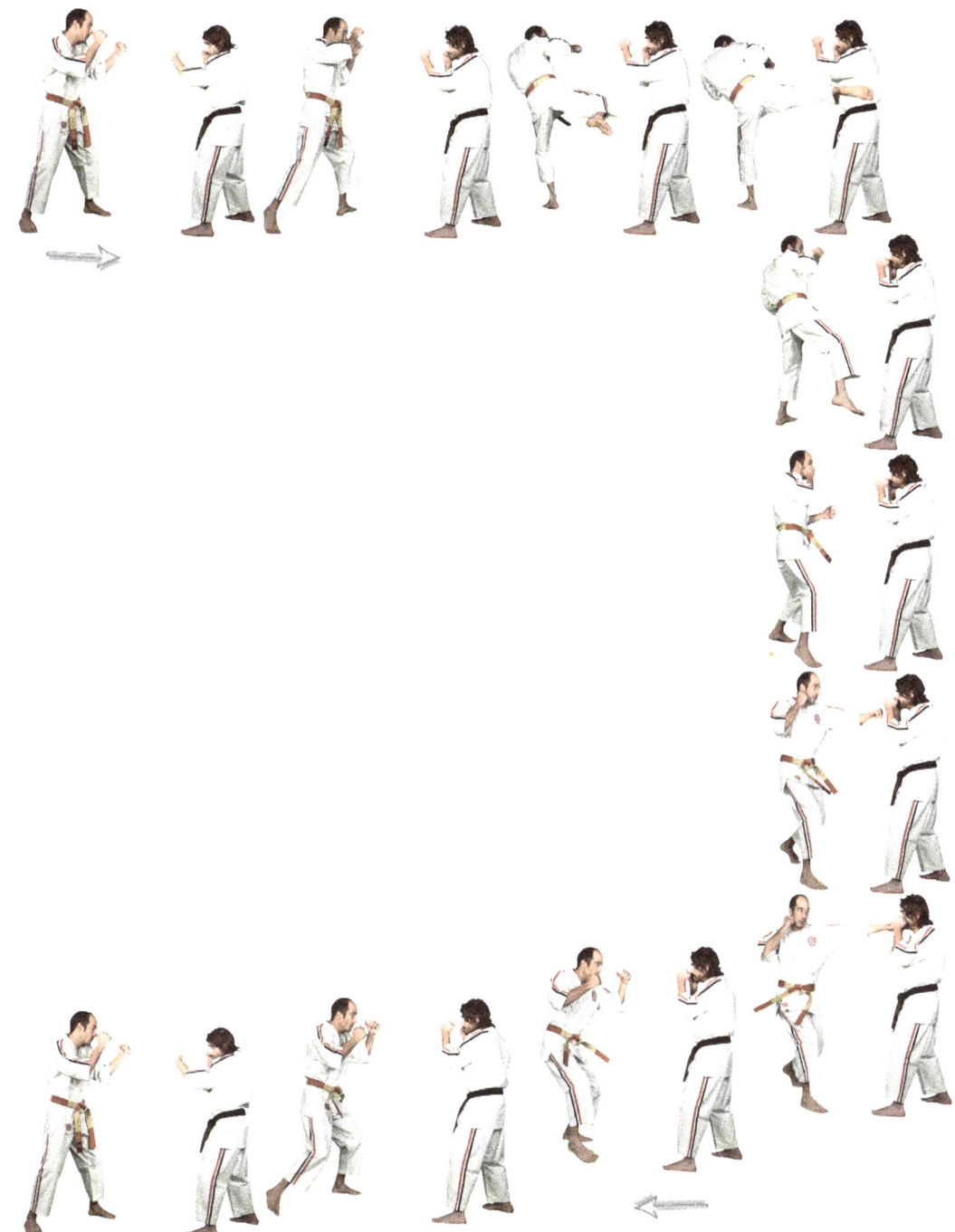

Figure 4.14: Combination of Two Techniques leading with Feet Combo 4.

Combo 5: From a left fighting stance, execute a left lunge front kick to the body level. Put the left foot down immediately and execute a right twist roundhouse kick to the head level. Note: It is important to quickly retract the straight kick and get it to the ground as fast as possible to minimize the time between the two kicks. See Figure 4.15 for a detailed illustration.

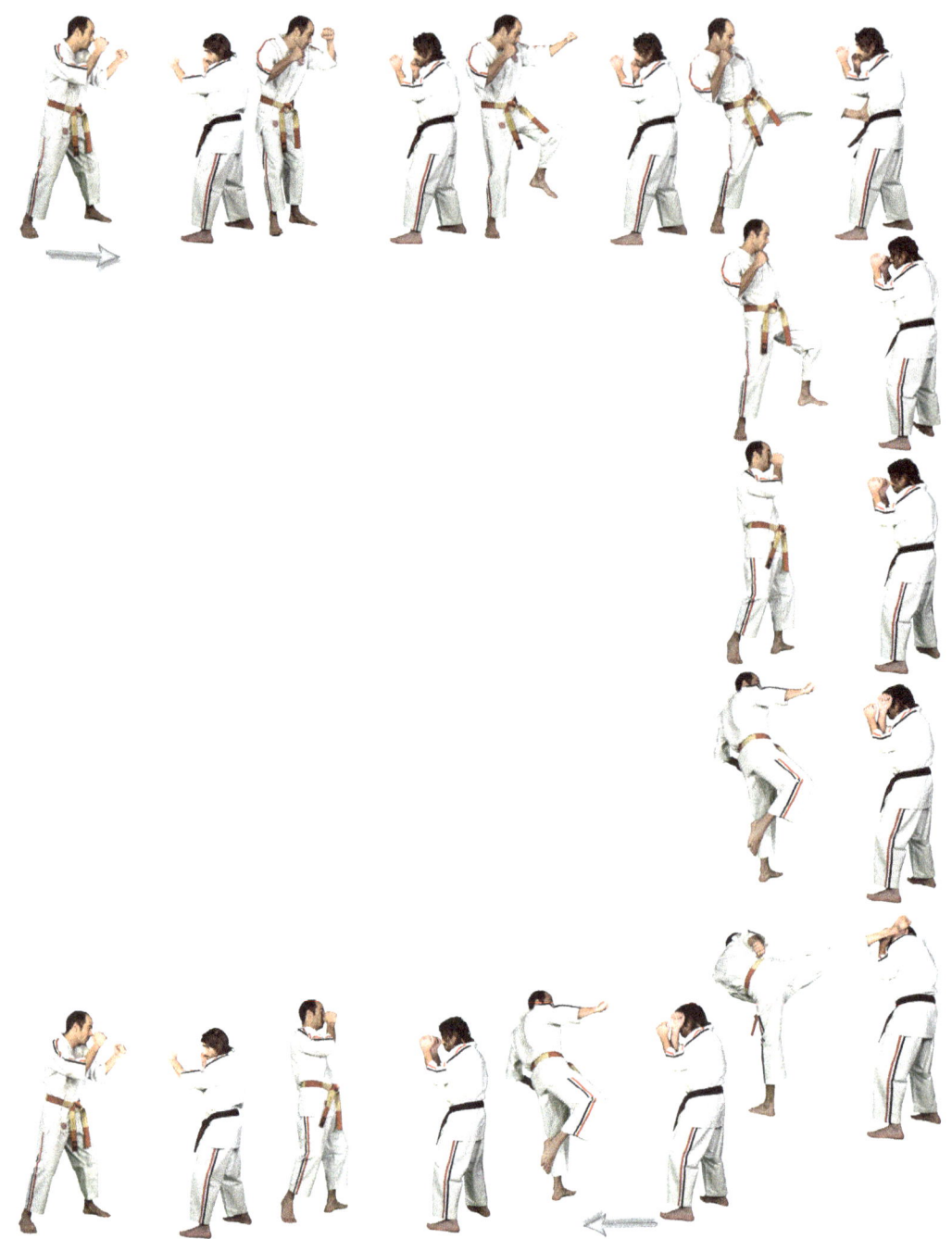

Figure 4.15: Combination of Two Techniques leading with Feet Combo 5.

Combo 6: From a left fighting stance, execute a right twist front kick to the body level. Put the right foot down immediately in a right fighting stance and execute a left Twist roundhouse kick to the head level. As in combo 5, it is important to make the transition between techniques as quick as possible by a quick retraction of the right straight kick. See Figure 4.16.

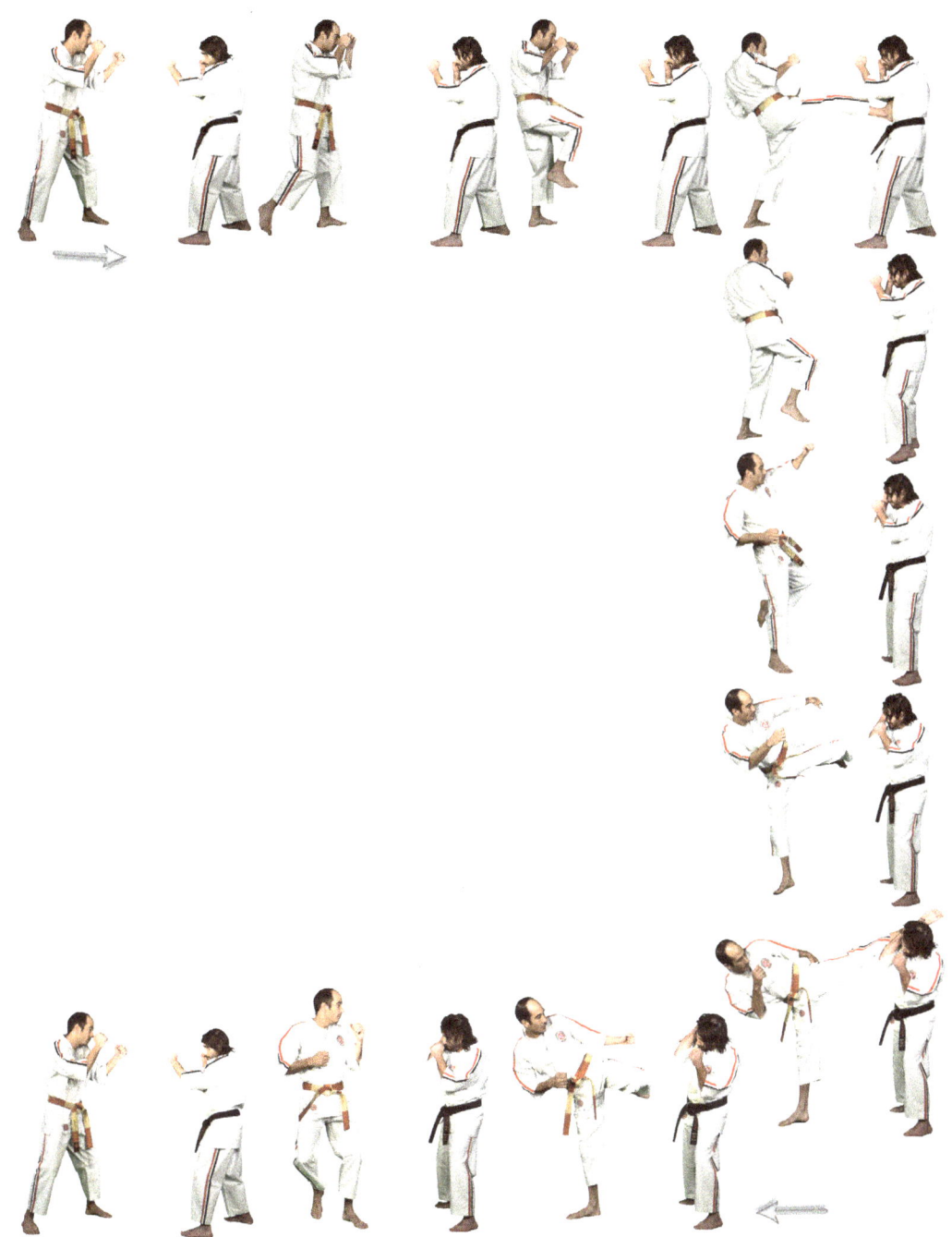

Figure 4.16: Combination of Two Techniques leading with Feet Combo 6.

Combo 7: From a left fighting stance, execute a right back roundhouse kick to the body level. Put the right foot down immediately in a right fighting stance and execute a left twist straight punch to the head level. See Figure 4.17.

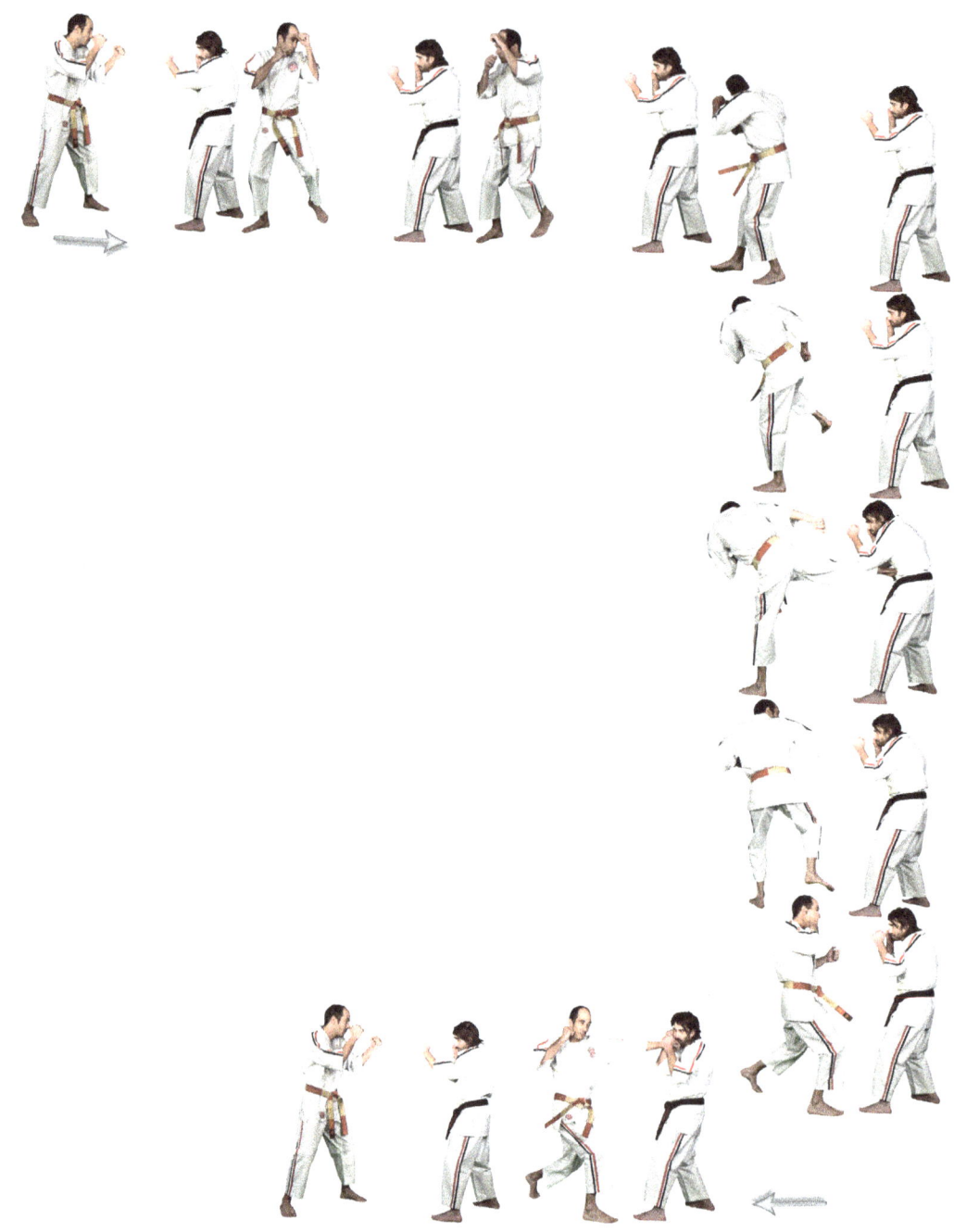

Figure 4.17: Combination of Two Techniques leading with Feet Combo 7.

4.7 THREE TECHNIQUES COMBINATION

4.7.1 LEADING WITH THE HANDS

Combo 8: From a left fighting stance, execute a left front straight punch to the head level, immediately followed by a right twist straight punch to the head level. Then execute a left roundhouse kick to the body level or lower level stepping with the right foot to adjust distance and step off the target line (slightly right). Note: The left punch could be substituted with a left hook punch or other suitable left-hand technique. See Figure 4.18.

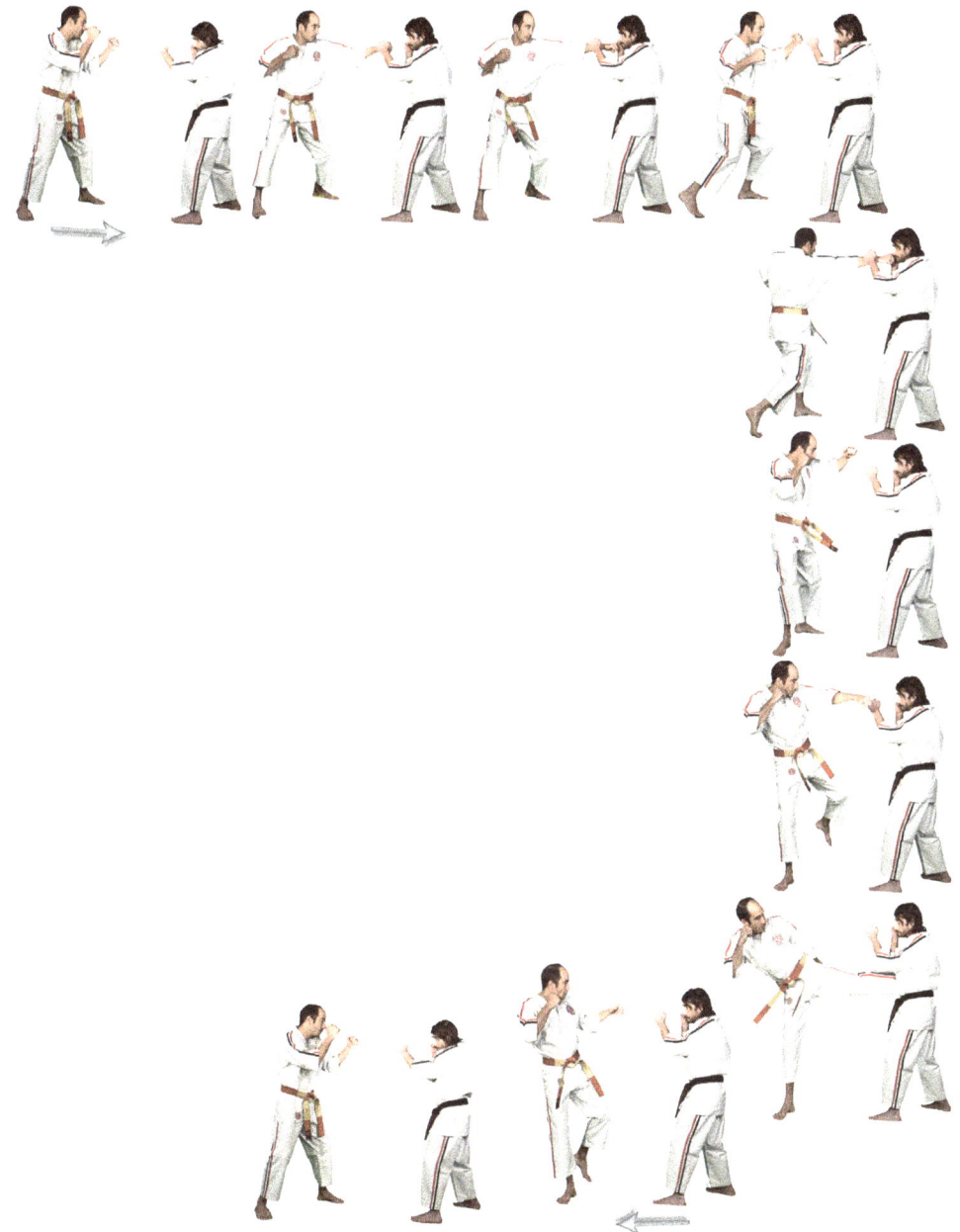

Figure 4.18: Combination of Three Techniques leading with Hands Combo 8.

Combo 9: From a left fighting stance, execute a right twist front punch to the head level immediately followed by a left front straight punch to the head level. Then execute a right twist roundhouse kick to the body level or lower level stepping with the left foot to adjust distance and step off the target line (slightly left). Note: As with combo 9, this combo can be practiced with a left hook punch or other left-hand technique. See Figure 4.19.

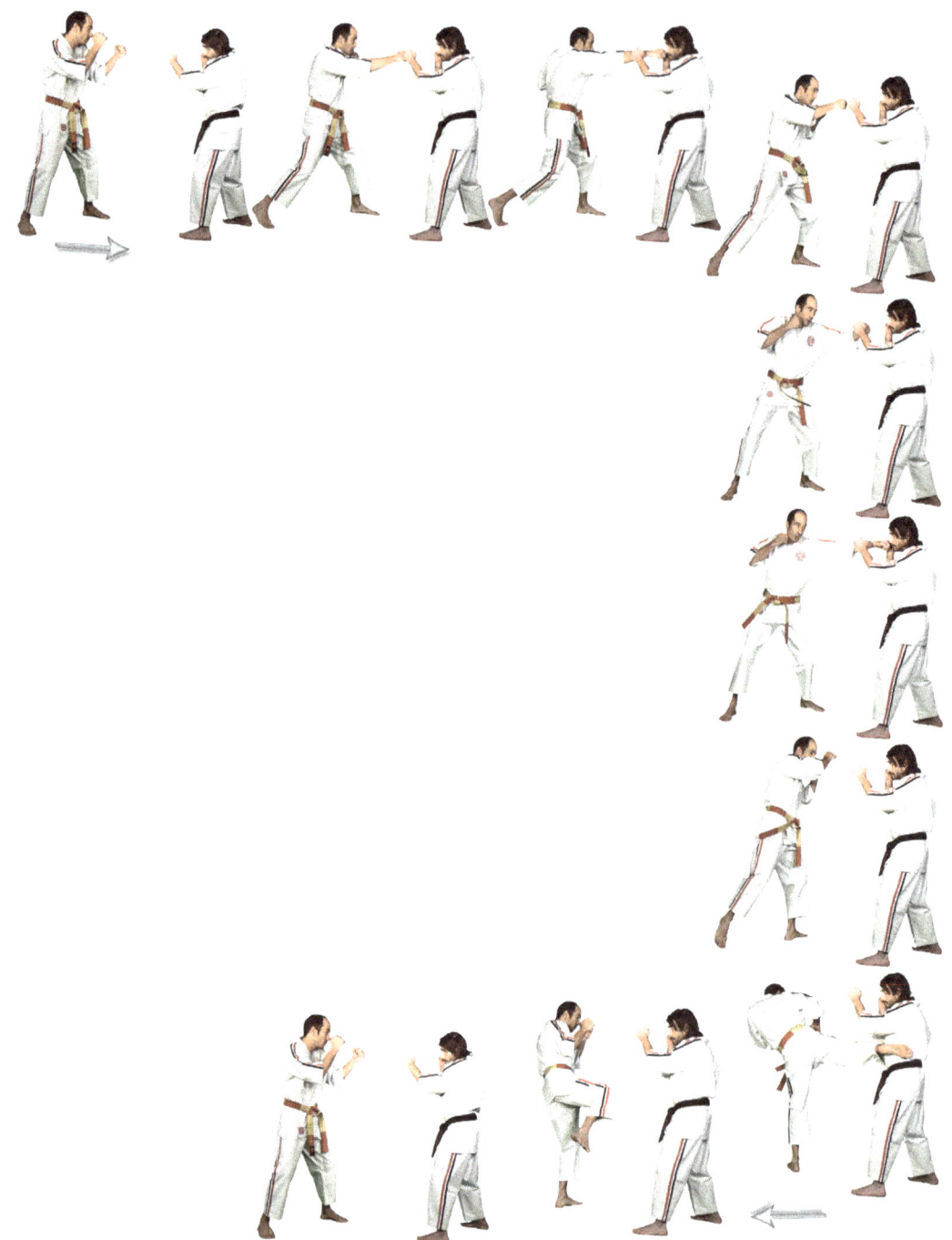

Figure 4.19: Combination of Three Techniques leading with Hands Combo 9.

4.7.2 LEADING WITH THE FEET

Combo 10: From a left fighting stance, execute a left lunge roundhouse kick to the body or lower level. Put the left foot down and execute a right twist straight punch to the head level followed by a left front straight punch to the head level. Note: Try substituting the left punch at the end of this combo with a hook punch or another left roundhouse kick to the body. See Figure 4.20.

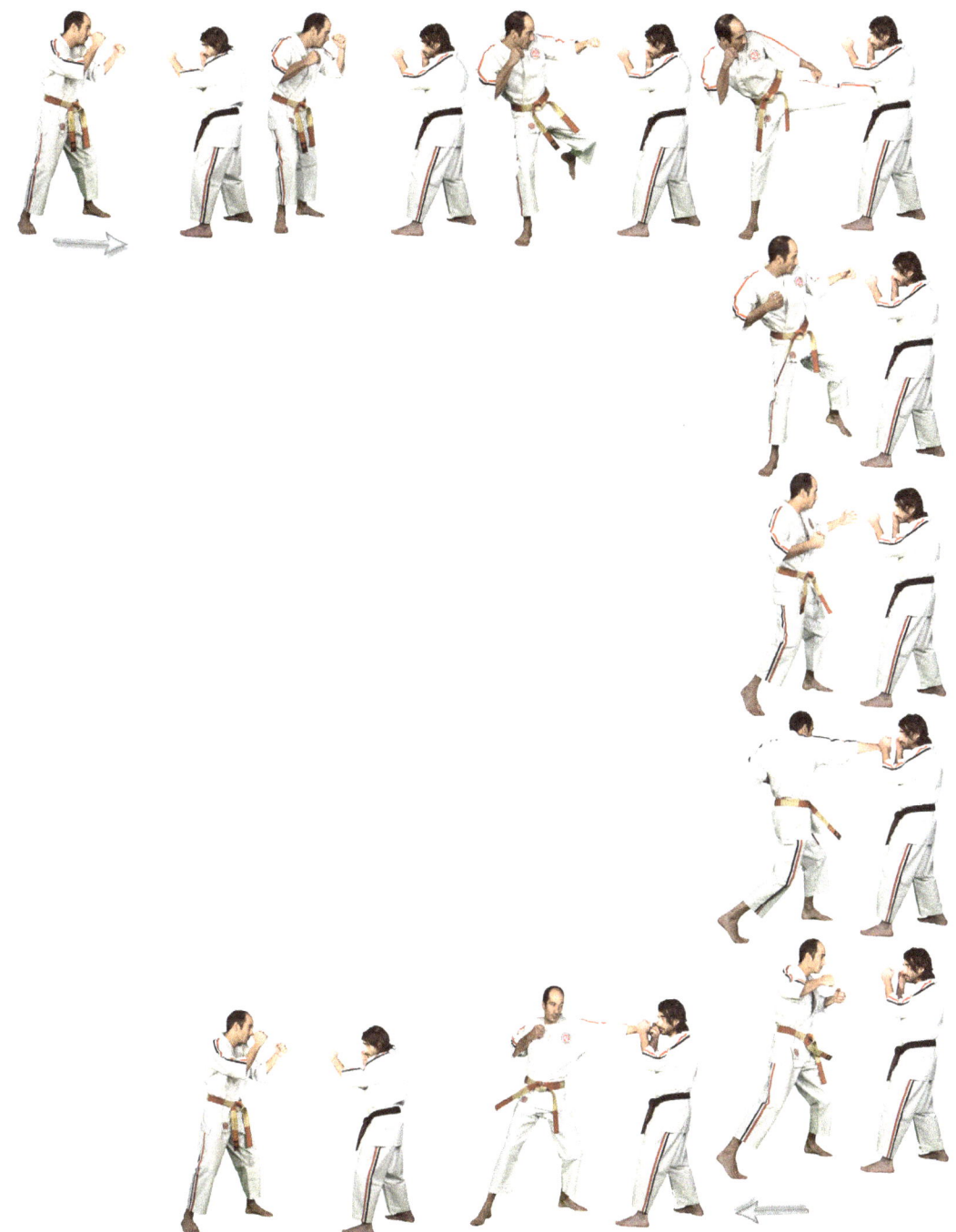

Figure 4.20: Combination of Three Techniques leading with Feet Combo 10.

Combo 11: From a left fighting stance, execute a right twist roundhouse kick. Put the right foot down immediately in a right fighting stance and execute a left Twist straight punch to the head level followed by a right front straight punch to the head level. Note: Try substituting the right front straight punch at the end of the combo with a right hook or another right roundhouse kick. If the distance increases or a right knee strike, should the opponent close the distance for a takedown or grabbing technique. See Figure 4.21.

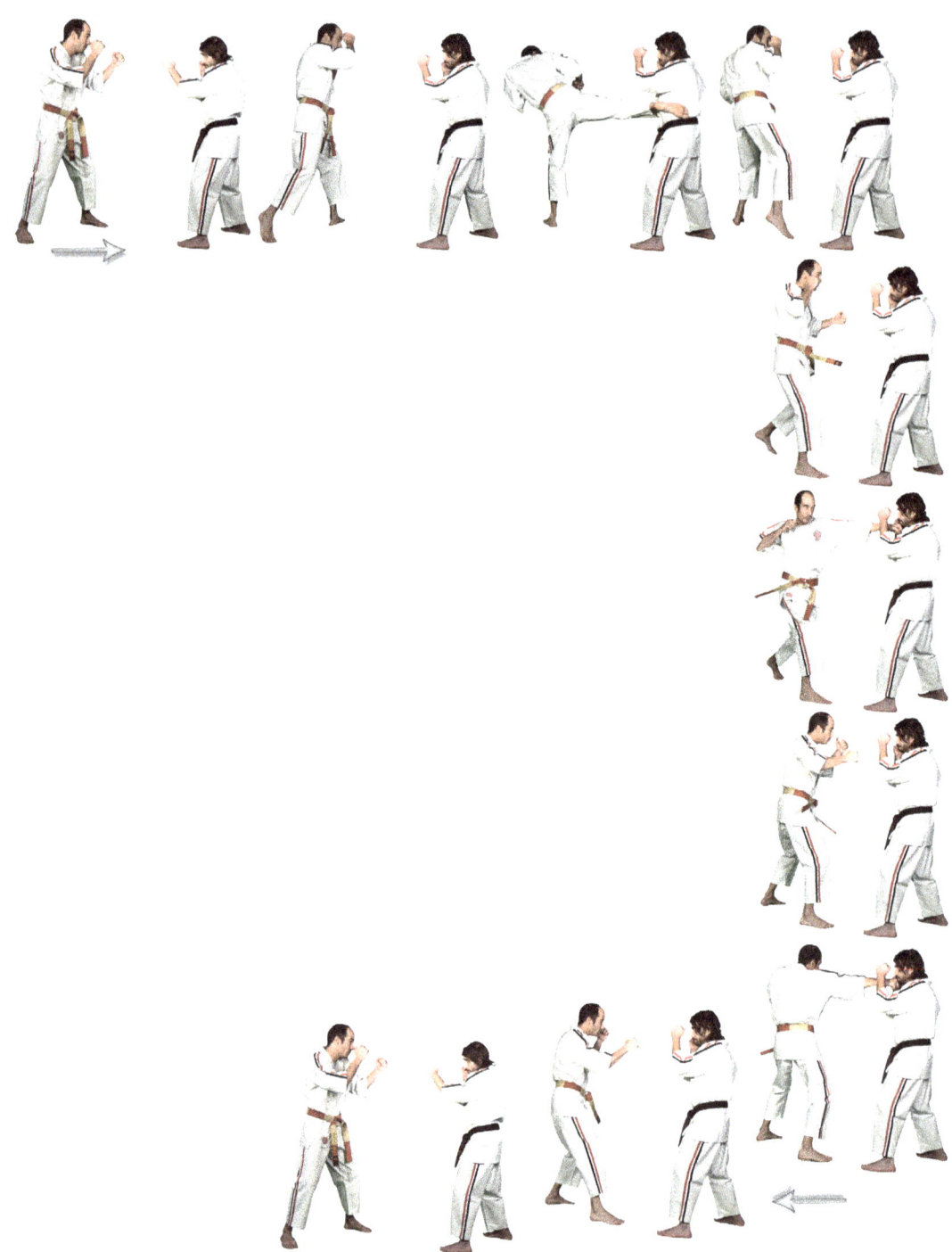

Figure 4.21: Combination of Three Techniques leading with Feet Combo 11.

Combo 12: From a left fighting stance, execute a left lunge front kick to the body level. Put the left foot down immediately and execute a right twist roundhouse kick to the body level. Put the right foot down in a right fighting stance and execute a left twist straight punch to the head level. See Figure 4.22.

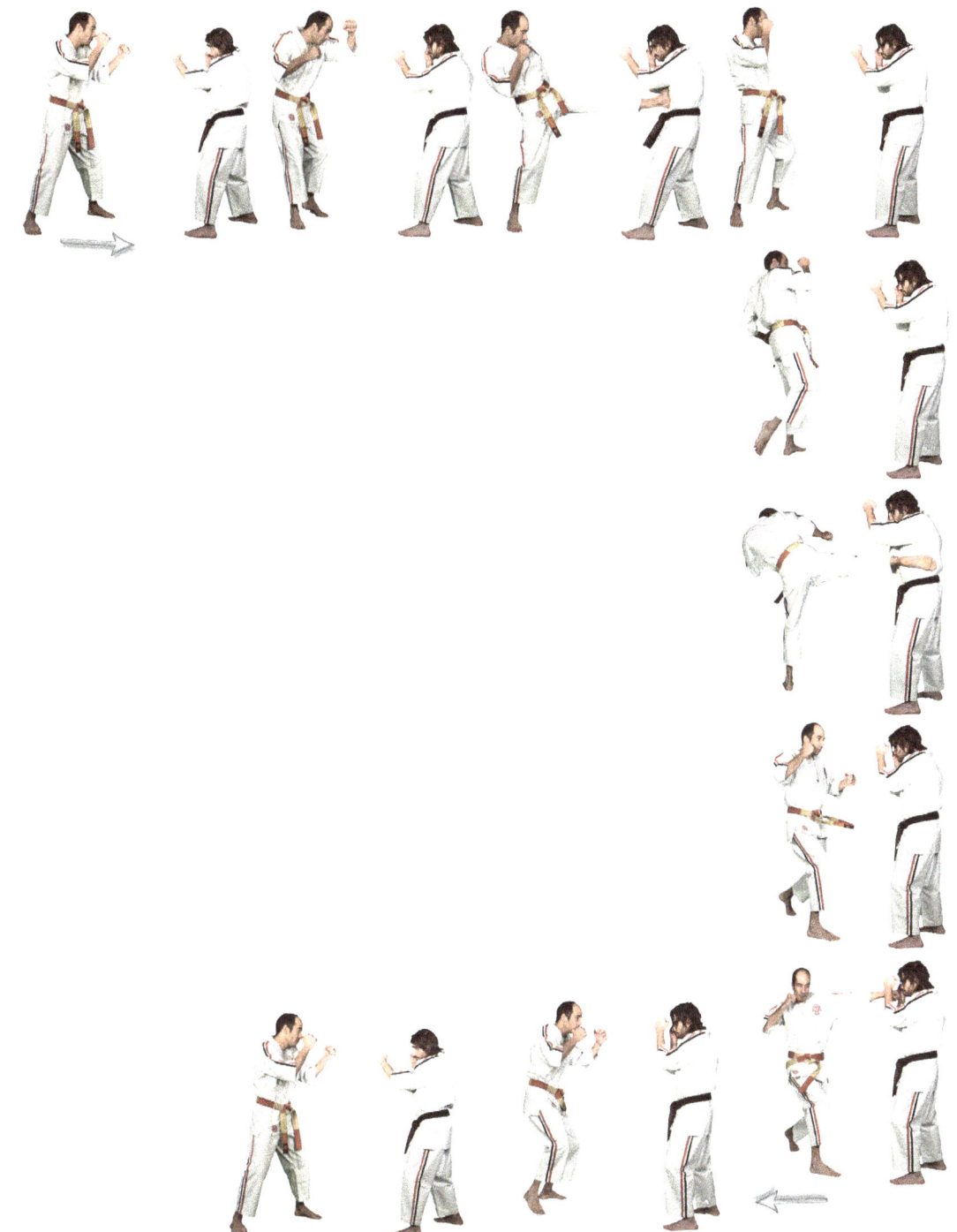

Figure 4.22: Combination of Three Techniques leading with Feet Combo 12.

Combo 13: From a left fighting stance, execute a right twist front kick to the body level. Put the right foot down immediately in a right fighting stance and execute a left twist roundhouse kick to the body level. Put the left foot down and execute a right twist straight punch to the head level. See Figure 4.23.

CHAPTER 4: OFFENSIVE FIGHTING | 123

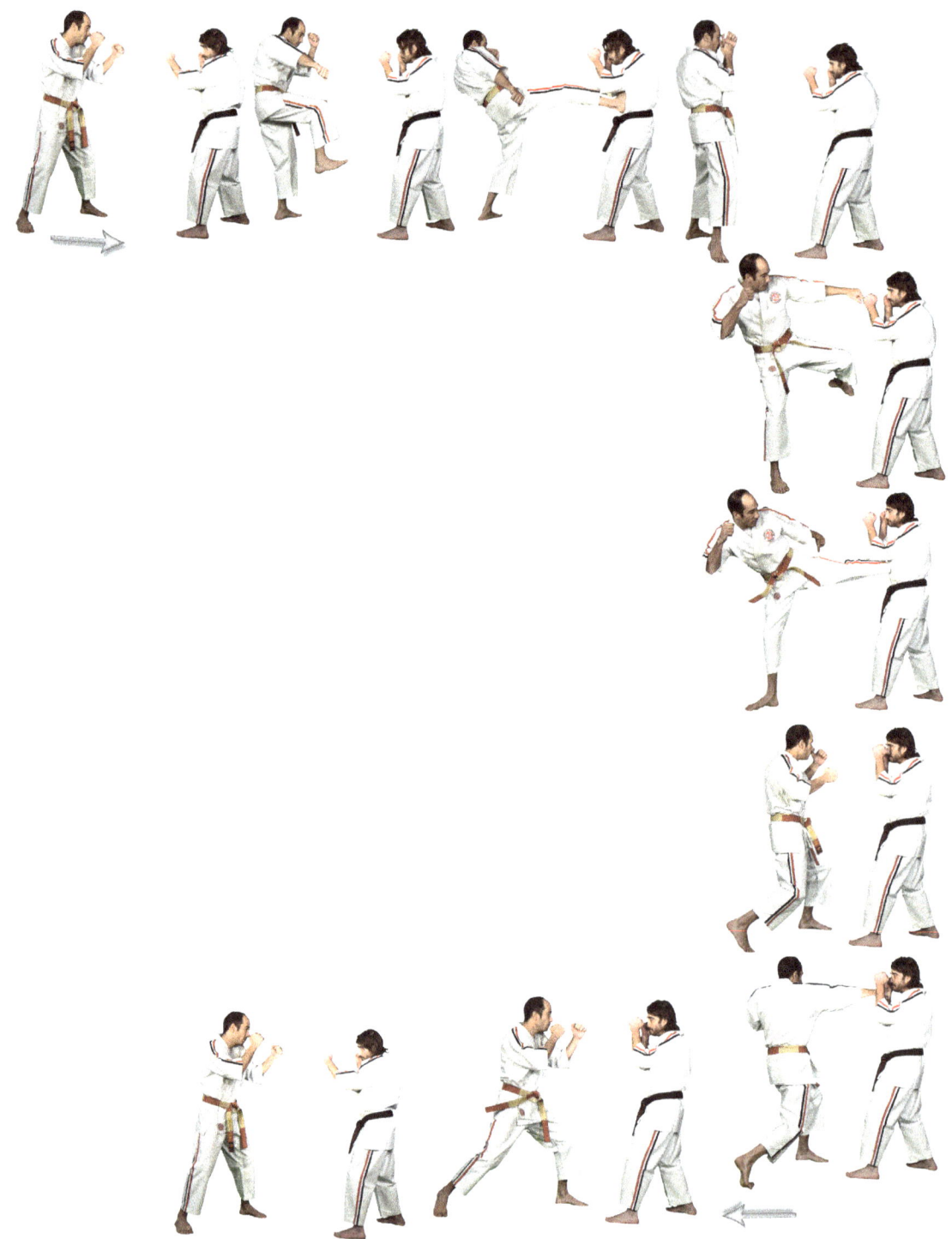

Figure 4.23: Combination of Three Techniques leading with Feet Combo 13.

Combo 14: From a left fighting stance, execute a left lunge side kick to the body level. Then quickly retract the side kick and place the foot to the ground slightly to the right of the target and execute a right back roundhouse kick to the body level. Put down the right foot immediately in a right fighting stance and execute a left twist straight punch to the head level. See Figure 4.24.

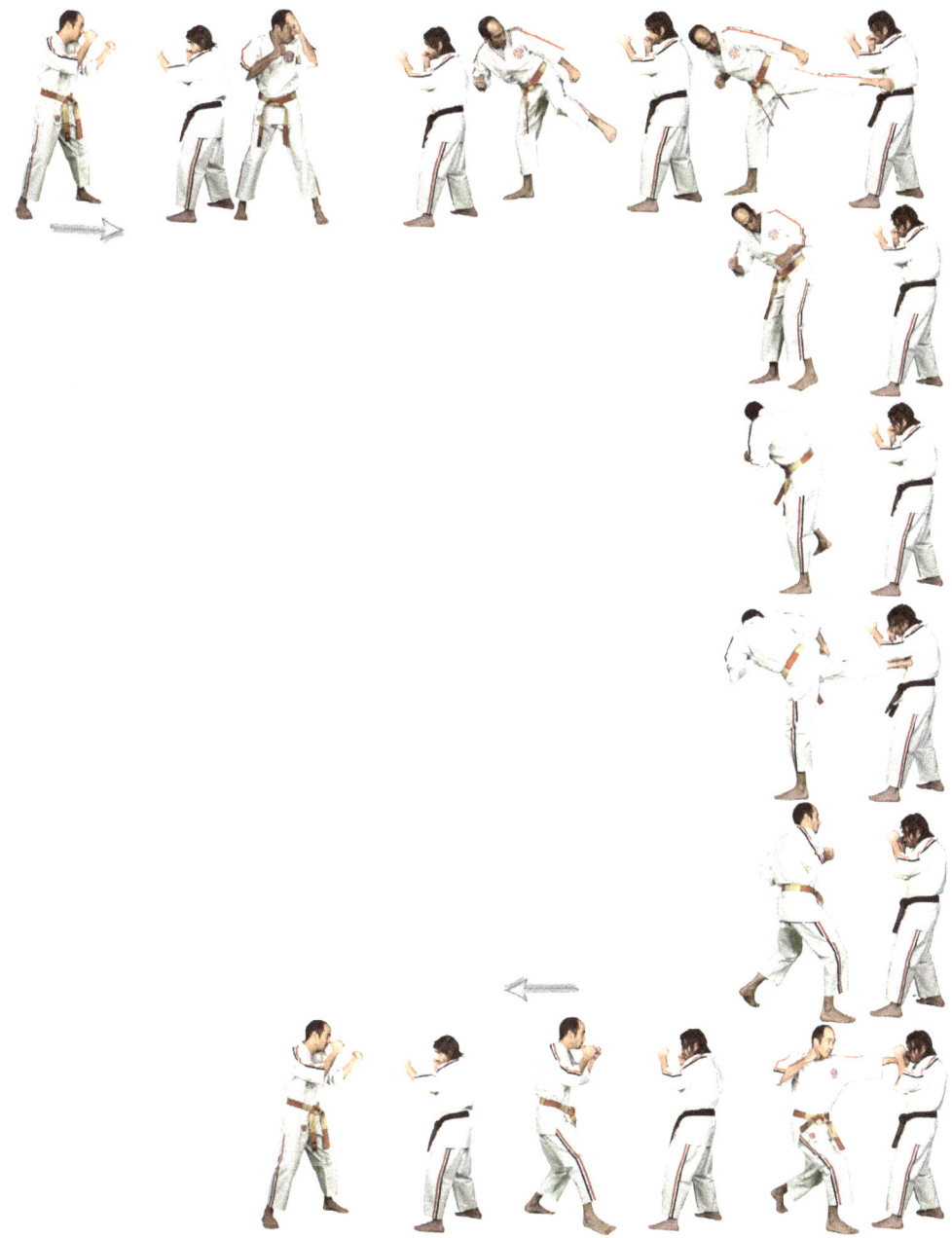

Figure 4.24: Combination of Three Techniques leading with Feet Combo 14.

Combo 15: From a left fighting stance, execute a right back-roundhouse kick to the body level. Put the right foot down immediately in a right fighting stance and execute a left twist straight punch to the head level followed by a right roundhouse kick to the body or lower level. The left foot is moved to adjust the distance for the kick and get off the target line (slightly left). See Figure 4.25.

As mentioned at the beginning of this section, there are limitless combinations that can be successfully used in self-defense and contact fighting. The 15 combinations described above form a basic foundation to understand how to formulate and tailor a combination using 2 or 3 techniques. Each combination caters to specific needs, such as changing distance and angles, and cutting off the opponent when implementing an offensive strategy.

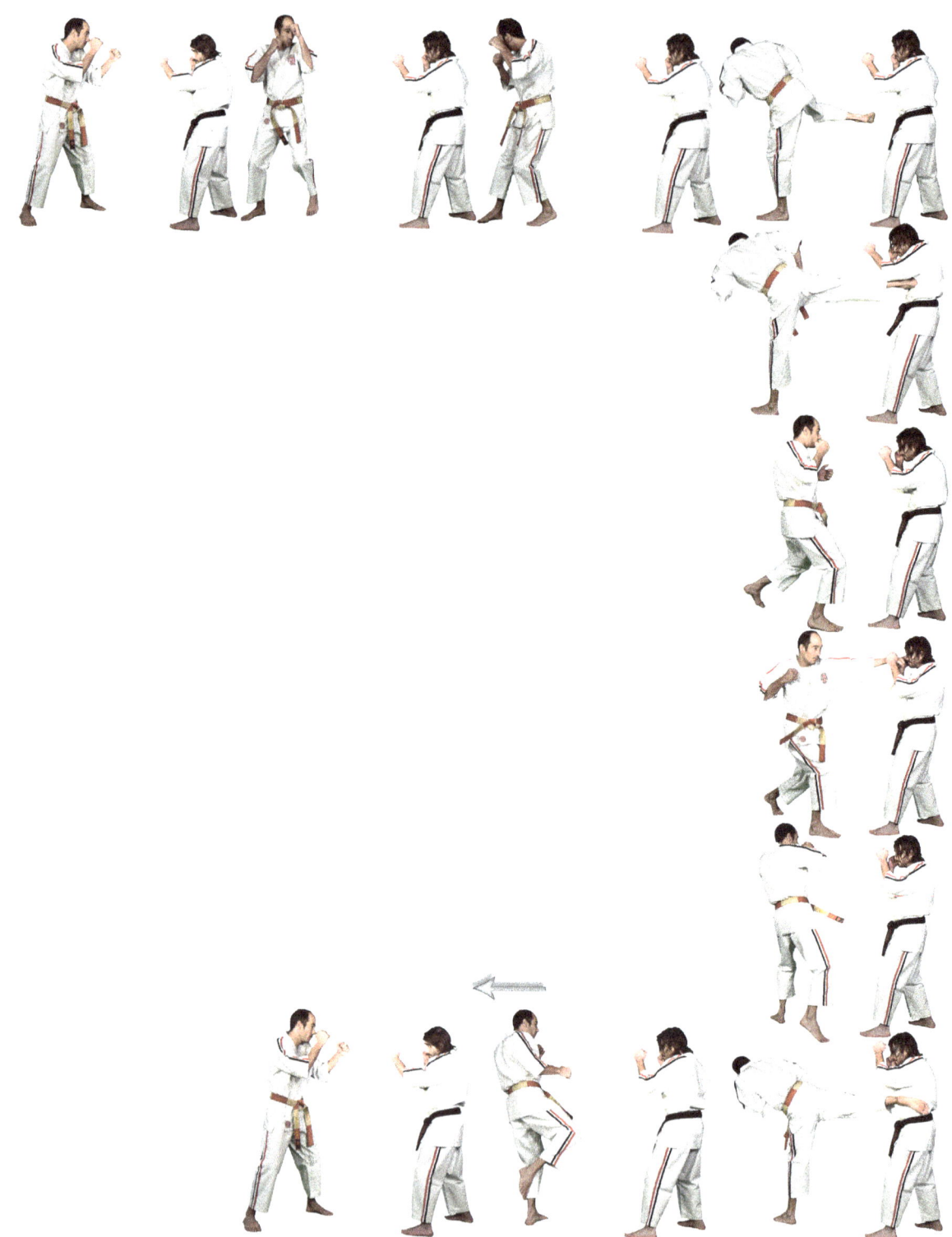

Figure 4.25: Combination of Three Techniques leading with Feet Combo 15.

CHAPTER 5: DEFENSIVE FIGHTING

THE CONCEPT OF defensive fighting involves allowing the opponent to initiate the attack with the intention of reacting to that attack with a counterattack. This strategy offers the fighter to anticipate the location of the target at the moment of execution. By using this strategy, one knows exactly where one's opponent is because they are committed due to their attack. While there are many ways to achieve an opportunity to counterattack, one of the most effective way is to utilize some form of movement to escape the opponent's attack and places oneself in a position to counterattack. Besides movement there are blocking and covering techniques that can be used to absorb an attack before countering the attack. The traditional karate strategy is of escape and counter, mainly because karate was originally developed to defend against attacks with swords. The other factor to think about is the size and strength of the opponent. It is unfavorable to attempt to absorb the attacks before countering by the bigger or stronger opponent as there is likelihood that one may lose balance or get injured by the attack. For this reason, it is preferable to escape than to block or cover up, and it can be used to allow a counterattack either after or at the same time or even slightly before the opponent's attack. It is important to understand that defensive movements do not help in winning a fight and so it must always be accompanied by a counterattack. It is important to develop the strategy to escape at the right distance neither over escaping and making the distance too far to counter, nor under escaping and ending up facing further attacks.

The good defensive skill consists of examining and developing an understanding of footwork or movement, timing of counter, deflecting or blocking techniques and selection of counter techniques. This chapter will look at the different methods for escaping and the different times for counterattack along with their applications and the selection of techniques for countering different attacks.

5.1 ESCAPING ON THREE LEVELS

The basic purpose of escaping techniques is to avoid an incoming attack and a counterattack technique can be used. This can be accomplished in 3 different ways which can be used on their own or combined together. These three ways of escaping are foot, body, and head, and are usually done in that order.

The escaping by foot is done by stepping and moving the whole body to dodge the oncoming attack. There are several different steps that can be used and will be discussed later in this chapter. The escaping using body movement is done by shifting the body weight from one leg to the other and shifting the upper body over that leg. This shifting of the body is usually done in a backward direction or can be done side to side to dodge incoming attack. The escaping using head movement is done by shifting the shoulders and head back, side to side or downward by bending the knees. These three ways of escaping should be done simultaneously one after another allowing 3 opportunities to escape the attack. In case the foot movement isn't enough, the body movement might be enough, and if the foot and body movement aren't enough then the head movement may still slip the technique. It is also advised to combine these 3 levels of escaping with a deflecting or blocking technique which serves as an extra level of escaping and can also create an off balanced moment for the attacking opponent. It will give an opportunity to grab the opponent or catch their technique to execute a sweeping or throwing technique.

5.2 FOOT MOVEMENT

There are several different ways and directions that one can use to escape an attack and create an opportunity to counterattack. The preferable directions are the ones that not only escape the attack but also get oneself off the attack line requiring the opponent to redirect in another direction. For this purpose, the main escaping directions are focused on 45 degrees angle backward or forward, and also sometimes straight in to the opponent usually when executing a simultaneous or pre-emptive counter strike. It is important to note that 45 degrees angle is a starting point and it must be adjusted depending on the height and effective range of the opponent. The 45 degrees angle of escape is used when facing an opponent of equal height and reach, increase that angle close to 90 degrees as the opponent's height and reach increases. For a much taller opponent escaping at almost 90 degrees or laterally is preferred, this will help to stifle the reach of the opponent and keep oneself within an achievable striking distance. Likewise, when facing a shorter opponent, the escape angle should be less and close to escaping directly backward. In this way, the shorter opponent is kept at a further distance and allows one to take advantage of the range difference. With this understanding of 45 degrees escape, the following escape forms will be described, however, they should be practiced with opponents of different heights to learn to adjust the angle of escape as necessary.

5.3 ESCAPE FORMS

5.3.1 NEKO ASHI (CAT STEP ESCAPE, FRONT SIDE ESCAPE)

From left fighting stance, push the left foot stepping backwards while placing the right foot at an angle of approximately 45 degrees to the attack line. In addition to stepping, make sure the body adjusts for the changing direction so that it remains centered to the target and able to counter effectively. The left foot should follow the step and reposition it in a balanced stance centered to the opponent. This escaping motion is aided by shifting the body weight slightly over the right foot in a form of back stance. It can also be aided by a deflecting technique with either hand, to deflect an attack to the left which is basically in the opposite direction one is stepping in. This escape technique can also be used with the hands and arms covering the face and vitals, similar to boxing and other large gloved fighting competitions. See Figure 5.1 and video for detailed illustrations.

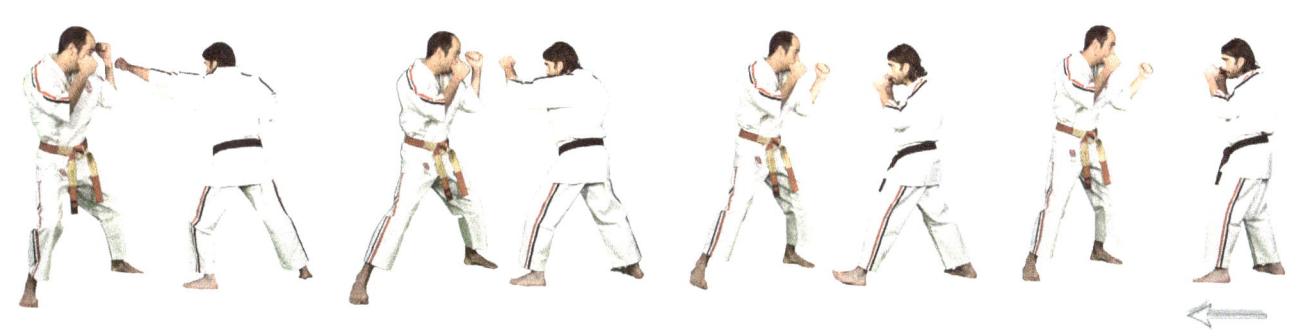

Figure 5.1: Illustration of Neko Ashi showing cat step escape and front side escape.

5.3.2 HIRAKI ASHI (OPEN LEG STEP, TURNING ESCAPE)

From left fighting stance, push the right foot pivoting on the left foot, turning the hips and shoulders in a clockwise direction. When the body has turned to an approximately 45 degrees angle, step back with the right foot and place it in a left fighting stance, centered to the target and at 45 degrees angle to the original attack line. In the above escape form, the left foot may need to be repositioned to achieve a balanced and centered stance. Additionally, as with the Neko Ashi escape form described above, the body weight can be shifted to a back stance to create a further escaping motion. This can also be aided by using the hands in a deflecting and blocking technique or by covering up with the hands and arms. See Figure 5.2 and video.

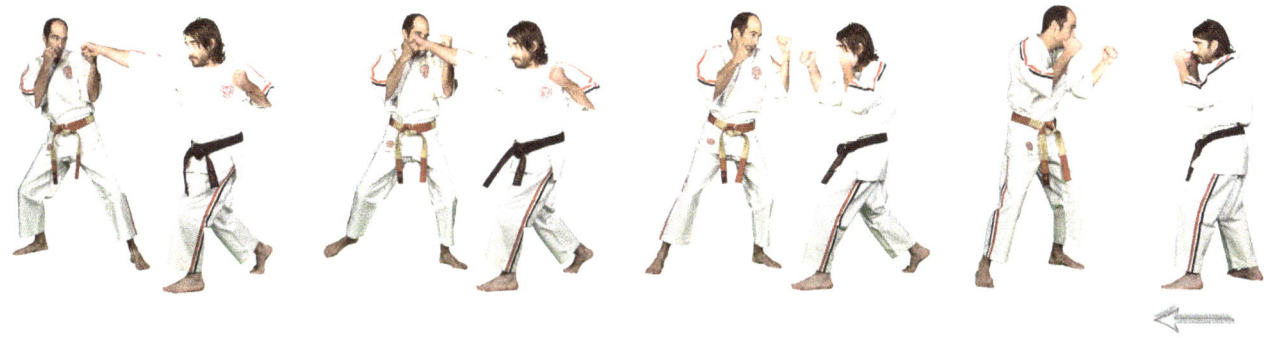

Figure 5.2: Illustration of Hiraki Ashi showing Open Leg Step and Turning Escape.

5.3.3 OI ASHI (LUNGE ESCAPE, SWITCHING ESCAPE)

From left fighting stance, push the left foot and step backwards placing the left foot close to the right foot and at an angle of 45 degrees to the attack line. By adopting a right fighting stance, it should be centered to the target and at 45 degrees angle to the original fighting stance. This can be combined with body shift, deflecting and blocking technique or cover with hands and arms as with other escape forms. See Figure 5.3 and video.

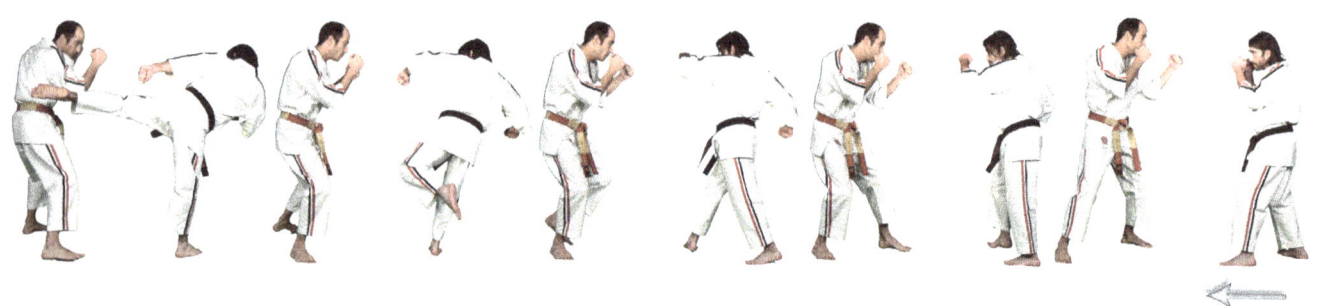

Figure 5.3: Illustration of Oi Ashi showing Lunge Escape and Switching Escape.

5.3.4 SANKAKU ASHI (TRIANGLE STEP)

From a left fighting stance, push off the right foot and take a small step forward and placing the left foot at 45 degrees angle to the attack line (left of the target). Immediately follow the left foot with the right foot, and place it behind the left foot while turning the hips and shoulders to be centered to the target. Then push off the right foot and step forward towards the target with the left foot, and at the same time execute the counter technique as the last step. This stepping motion forms a triangle with the original line of attack. This escaping motion is particularly useful in situations where there is no room to move backwards at angle and one must move forward. It is mainly used for delivering counter attacks and for maneuvering towards opponent's back simultaneously.

To perform this form of escape by moving to the right, step with the right foot forward and 45 degrees to the right of the target. Then follow the right foot with the left foot and place it behind the right foot while turning counter clockwise the hips and shoulders should be centered to the target. Right away push off the left foot and step forward toward the target with the right foot in a right fighting stance or forward stance, execute the chosen counter technique or grappling position. See Figure 5.4 and video.

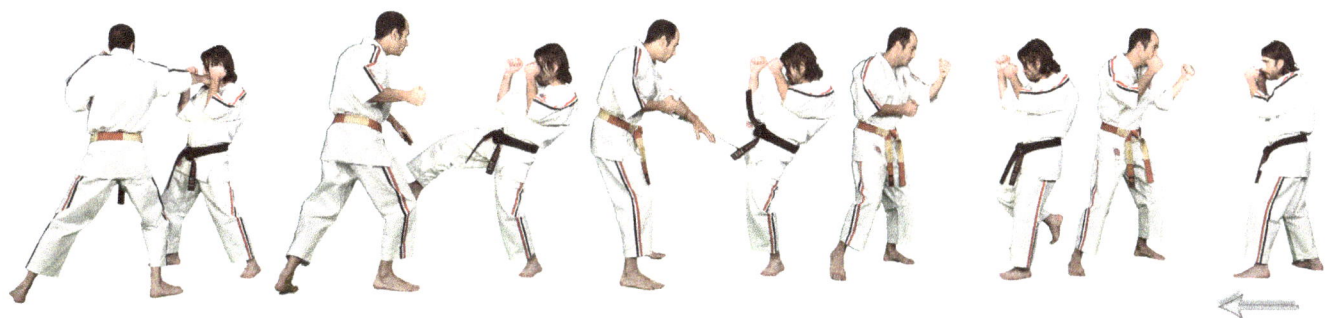

Figure 5.4: Illustration of Sankaku Asi sowing Triangle Step.

5.3.5 STRAIGHT IN ESCAPE

Circular techniques such as roundhouse kicks, hook punches and other circular striking techniques offer an opportunity to be "stepped-in on" as they have to travel a farther distance than a straight technique. This basic principal allows the opportunity to escape by moving straight in and attacking. This technique is used effectively to execute pre-emptive and simultaneous counter attacks against circular attacks.

From a left fighting stance, push off the right foot stepping with the left foot straight forward towards the opponent, either immediately executing the counterstrike which is usually a straight punch or kick, or grabbing the opponent for a throwing, sweeping or take down technique. See Figure 5.5 and video.

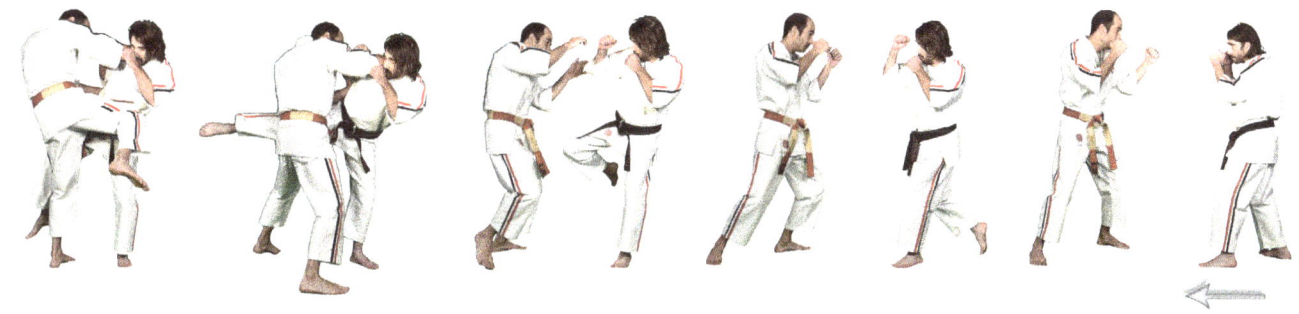

Figure 5.5: Illustration of the Straight in Escape Technique

5.4 SELECTING ESCAPING MOTIONS AND ANGLES

The choice of escape form largely depends upon the characteristics of the opponent one is facing. In general, there are only few types of opponents a fighter may have to face, they are the Taller, shorter, heavier and lighter opponent. Some opponents may possess 2 or more of these characteristics which may affect choice of movement.

When facing a taller opponent, the general strategy is to get into the comfortable range of the taller opponent where one can effectively execute the technique. But if the opponent is too close, one must maintain a larger distance outside the opponent range. For this purpose, the lunging step escape is highly recommended in conjunction with close to 50-80 degrees lateral angle. This escape form allows for the largest amount of distance to be covered and is good for changing directions quickly. The turning step escape is recommended against taller opponents which allows to quickly change directions and getting off the attack line while maintaining a close range. Another effective strategy for taller opponents is the straight in escape, taking advantage of the opponent throwing a roundhouse kick from either leg.

While facing the shorter opponent, the general strategy of a longer reach must be utilized to keep the opponent at a distance which is just out of range for them. For this purpose, Cat step escape and the turning step escape are emphasized in conjunction with 15-35 degrees angle close to straight back. This way it is possible to maintain a larger range.

While facing the heavier opponent, the general strategy is to stay off the attack line and maintain a comfortable counter distance to avoid the power directly in front of the heavier opponent. The quick moveable footwork is required that can change directions when required. For this purpose, lunging escape, turning escape and triangle escape are recommended.

While facing the lighter opponent, the general strategy is to cut off the opponent's movement and prevent them from creating distance to slip and escape. For this purpose, straight in escape, small cat step and turning escapes are recommended. This will allow to maintain a closer range and make it easier to cut off the opponent's movement.

5.5 SELECTING COUNTER TECHNIQUES

The selection of right counterattack technique is extremely important as it will ultimately determine the success of the counterattack. When implementing a defensive strategy, there are three important things that need to be considered - escape technique, counter technique, and the timing to use. As discussed in the previous section, the type of escape motion depends upon the opponent's characteristics and the distance need to be maintained. Similarly, the selection of counter technique largely depends upon the distance, but in this case the distance of the opponent's attack. It is also based on the direction of the attack and shares very similar concepts as the formulation of combinations as discussed in the chapter on offensive fighting. In this way, counter techniques can be selected based on the following criteria:

5.5.1 COUNTERING WITH A DIFFERENT WEAPON

This refers to use of a hand technique to counter foot techniques and use of foot techniques to counter hand techniques. This method is very effective because it delivers the counter strike at a different distance than the opponent's attack and thus reducing the risk of being hit by the attack while attempting to counter strike.

5.5.2 COUNTERING WITH A DIFFERENT DIRECTION

This refers to counter attacking from a different direction than the opponent's attack. The straight technique is used to counter a round technique and vice versa. By changing the direction, it allows the fighter to deliver a counter strike while changing position or angle it also reduces the risk of getting hit by the attack or follow-up attack.

5.5.3 COUNTERING AT A DIFFERENT LEVEL

This refers to executing the counterattack technique at a different target than the opponent's attack, i.e. counter attacking at lower or middle level when attacked at the upper level and counter attacking at the upper level when attacked at the middle or lower level. This method will increase the chances of landing the counterattack technique and decrease the instances of other techniques from being clashed.

By using one or more of these criteria's when selecting techniques for counterattack, one can increase their chances of both avoiding the attack and landing the counterattack.

5.6 TIMING: GONOSEN, TAINOSEN AND SENNOSEN (POST ATTACK, SIMULTANEOUS ATTACK AND PRE-EMPTIVE ATTACK)

The idea of timing for defensiveness refers to the moment in which one can execute a counterattack in relation to the opponent's attack. In this way, it is possible to execute a counterattack at one of 3 different times, just after the attack, simultaneous to the attack or at the same time, and just before the beginning of the attack.

5.6.1 GONOSEN: COUNTERING AFTER THE ATTACK (POST ATTACK)

This counterattack timing involves counter attacking just after the opponent has executed their attack. It requires the use of an escape motion or covering and blocking motion to nullify the opponents attack followed by quick execution of the counterattack. This type of timing is favorable when facing a shorter opponent and or heavier opponent who may be slightly slower in movement and attack. However, it could be disadvantageous against a faster and more agile opponent, mainly because they may be able to escape after their attack faster than the counterattack. This counterattack timing can also be disadvantageous against a taller opponent where the distance is too far to cover after the attack and one may get stuck just outside the range.

The strategies for timing utilizing Tainosen and Sennosen are recommended against these types of opponents.

5.6.2 TAINOSEN: COUNTERING AT THE SAME TIME OF THE ATTACK (SIMULTANEOUS)

This counterattack timing involves executing the counterattack at the same time as the opponent attack. It requires the use of an escape motion in conjunction with the counterattack. In this way, it utilizes the movement used to execute the counterattack as the escaping motion. It also allows to strike and escape at the same time. The selection of proper technique is essential when executing a Tainosen counterattack. By using an inappropriate technique, it can result in an ineffective counterattack and possibly getting hit by the attack. Tainosen is recommended when facing either a taller or faster opponent, as it allows to execute the counterattack when one is sure that the opponent cannot escape because they are committed to their attack. This makes it harder for a quick agile opponent to slip and evade the counter attacks or for a taller opponent to keep distance.

5.6.3 SENNOSEN: COUNTERING JUST BEFORE THE ATTACK (PRE-EMPTIVE)

This counterattack timing is the most advanced form of timing because it involves identifying the moment that the opponent is about to execute attack, and counter attacking at the same moment. This type of timing technique is used with the straight in escape and mainly utilizes straight attacking techniques. In this technique, one moves forward, breaking the distance and landing into counterattack position while the opponent is in the mid execution of their attack.

This timing technique is known as Sannosen and recommended when fighting with taller and more powerful opponents. It allows the fighter to maintain adequate distance and pace and overcome the opponent's reach and power.

It is important to train and practice all 3 types of counterattack timing techniques for each of the major hand and foot attacks. By practicing the different types of timing techniques, one will be able to identify the opportunities for their application and the strategies for using them to overcome the strengths of the opponent. The table below shows some suggestions for selection of counterattack techniques based on the different escape motions and timing. See video for demonstration of these counters and timings.

TABLE 5.1 ATTACKING TECHNIQUES AND SUGGESTED COUNTER ATTACKING TECHNIQUES

Attacking Technique	Suggested Gonosen (post attack) Counter and escape	Suggested Tainosen (simultaneous to attack) Counter and escape	Suggested Sennosen (premptive to attack) Counter and escape
Choku Tsuki Straight punch, Jab or punch with the lead hand)	1. Twist punch to the head with Cat step escape. 2. Lead roundhouse kick to the body with Cat step escape.	1. Lead roundhouse kick to the body or leg with cat step escape. 2. Twist roundhouse kick to the leg with Cat step escape.	1. Lunge Front kick to the body with moving in escape.
Hineri Tsuki twist punch, reverse punch, cross or punch with the back hand	1. Twist punch to the head with turning step escape. 2. Twist roundhouse kick with turning escape.	1. Twist roundhouse kick with Lunging escape. 2. Ridge hand strike with cat step escape.	1. Twist Front kick with moving in escape.
Oi Mae Geri lunge front kick, straight kick with the front foot	1. Twist punch to the head with Cat step escape. 2. Twist roundhouse kick to the leg with Cat step escape.	1. Back Roundhouse kick with turning escape. 2. Spinning back Knife hand strike/Backfist with turning escape.	1. Straight punch or Jab with moving in escape. Punch can be substituted with a straight elbow for closer range applications.
Hineri Mae Geri twist front kick, straight kick with the back foot	1. Ridge hand strike with Turning escape. 2. Twist punch to the head with Cat step escape.	1. Twist Front kick (groin or body) with cat step escape. 2. Lunge front knife hand strike (right) with Triangle Step escape.	1. Twist punch to the head with moving in escape. Punch can be substituted with a straight elbow for closer range applications.
Oi Mawashi Geri lunge roundhouse kick, roundhouse kick with the front leg	1. Twist punch (left) with lunge step escape. 2. Straight punch or jab with turning escape.	1. Back Roundhouse kick with turning escape. 2. Spinning back Knife hand strike/Backfist with turning escape.	1. Straight punch or Jab with moving in escape. Punch can be substituted with a straight elbow for closer range applications.
Hineri Mawashi Geri twist roundhouse kick, swing round house kick, roundhouse kick with the back leg	1. Twist punch to the head with Cat step escape. 2. Twist Front kick with Cat step escape	1. Straight punch or Jab (right) with Triangle Step escape. 2. Lunge front kick(right) with triangle step escape.	1. Twist punch to the head with moving in escape. 2. Twist Front kick with moving in escape.

Ushiro Mawashi Geri Back roundhouse kick, spinning back kick, back wheel kick	1. Twist front knife hand strike with turning step escape. 2. Twist Roundhouse kick (left) with Lunging step escape	1. Twist front kick to the groin with turning escape.	1. Straight punch or Jab with moving in escape. 2. Front back chop (fist) with moving in escape.
Yoko Geri side kick	1. Straight punch or Jab with Cat step escape. 2. Spinning back Knife hand strike/Backfist with Cat step escape.	1. Straight punch or Jab (right) with Triangle Step escape.	1. Straight punch or Jab with moving in escape.

Note: All attacks and counter attacks in the above table are described as both fighters are in left fighting stance.

All counter attack techniques selection in the above table can be substituted with a similar technique for different distance. For example, kicks can be substituted for knee strikes of the same leg and punches can be substituted with elbow strikes or other strikes of the same hand for shorter range applications or dealing with opponents of dissimilar heights.

See Video for demonstration of all above countering techniques and timings

CHAPTER 6: STRATEGIES (PUTTING IT ALL TOGETHER)

THE BASIC TECHNIQUES and concepts for building strong and well-balanced striking techniques, and the concepts for offensive and defensive fighting, were discussed in the previous chapters. We will now look at putting together all the previous techniques and concepts and apply them in a strategic way to effectively overcome the opponent. Strategies can, therefore, be looked at as selecting the best movements, techniques, and timing to overcome the opponent. They involve identifying the opponent's strengths, weaknesses, favorite techniques, and preferred fighting style. By choosing the best movements, techniques, and timing, one can easily avoid opponent's strengths and exploit their weaknesses.

Strategies involve selection of different techniques or concepts such as, offensive or defensive, hand or foot techniques, straight or round techniques, movement, and timing. A good understanding of how to make these choices will help in developing the best strategies for any individual opponent.

6.1 OFFENSE VS DEFENSE

In general, whenever possible an offensive strategy is preferred over a defensive strategy, as the old saying goes "the best defense is a good offense". However, there are times when an offensive strategy may not be the best chance of victory. This is true in the case when facing a taller or larger opponent, or an opponent who has very good defensive counter attacking technique and footwork. In these situations, initiating the attack is not favorable, as it puts oneself against the strengths of the opponent. Offensive strategies can be utilized against a taller opponent however, one must be aware that the opponent will be looking for an opportunity to step in and close the distance to a more favorable range. When executing round or circular techniques, extra caution must be taken as they will offer the best opportunity for the opponent to step in. In this case, beginning with straight technique, then the use of combination technique is advised, followed by the round technique when the opponent is moving away.

Another strategy known as "Offensively defensive" strategy is very effective in situations where a straight offensive strategy fails. This strategy allows the fighter to move in an offensive way and still react defensively. In this strategy, the fighter moves forward posing to attack but waits for the opponent to attack in order to counterattack. This strategy is very effective at forcing a defensive opponent to attack, when they should rather be counter attacking. It is also good for cornering an opponent who is using footwork and movement to maintain a larger range.

6.2 HAND VS FOOT, STRAIGHT VS ROUND

When facing any opponent, a variety of hand and foot movements, straight and round techniques should be used. However, it is necessary at times to choose one or the other, especially, when selecting entry techniques for offensive attacks. When fighting with a shorter opponent, hand movements and straight techniques are preferable as entry techniques because they minimize the chances for the opponent to step in. Conversely, when facing a taller opponent, foot movements can help in closing the distance and round techniques will help with staying off the opponent's centerline and avoiding the opponent's reach and power.

6.3 MOVEMENT VS STANDING ONE'S GROUND OR STEPPING IN

Another strategy can be either to circle the opponent or to adopt a stationary rooted posture. A heavier or stronger opponent may be able to "run through" the smaller opponent if a planted or stationary posture is used. In this case, it is favorable to use circular movement prior to engaging in an attack. This will help to create an angle before attacking, allowing one to avoid their opponent's power. Conversely, when facing a lighter or faster opponent, a stationary rooted approach is used to implement a simultaneous or pre-emptive counter strike. Likewise, when facing a taller opponent, a stationary rooted posture strategy can be used so that one is ready to step in on the taller opponent to a more favorable range.

6.4 CHOOSING COUNTER TIMING

Another very important decision, when using a defensive or counter striking strategy is the counterattack timing. As discussed in the previous chapter, there are three different times at which a fighter can counter strike, after the attack, at the same time as the attack, and just before the attack. Choosing a preferred counter timing will depend on the characteristics of the opponent one is facing. In general, a taller or faster opponent will be able to use an "after the attack" counter timing very effectively as it allows them to maintain a greater distance and capitalize on an opponent that is having difficulty covering the extra range. Likewise, the shorter opponent will favor a more simultaneous or preemptive timing when stepping into an attack and to close the distance rather than escaping backwards and having a greater distance to cover for a counterattack. Similarly, the heavier or slower opponent must rely on simultaneous and pre-emptive counter timing to avoid being slightly short on range or slightly behind on timing. It is important to practice and train all three counterattack timings against all major attacking techniques to develop the most effective way to counterattack, depending on the opponent's strengths and favorite techniques.

6.5 SWITCHING OFFENCE AND DEFENSE

It is important to maintain the ability to switch between the strategies regardless of whether an offensive strategy or a defensive strategy is used. In other words, when attacking, one must be ready to switch to a defensive mode to defend oneself from the counterattack before switching back to offensive mode. A good example of this is, when one has stunned the opponent with an offensive technique and is going for the finish. At that moment, it is quite common for the opponent to lash out with an unexpected technique. In this situation, if one is too preoccupied with the offensive attack, then it is likely that one may get hit by an unexpected counter. Likewise, it is also important to become trained and practice switching from defensive mode to offensive mode. For example, when cornered it is advisable to counterattack without waiting for the opponent's attack. In this case, the best strategy is to switch to be offensive mode and attack. In this way, the opponent will be forced to deal with the attack, making space and time to get out of the corner. During that moment, the opponent is preoccupied with its own attack and isn't expecting the sudden switch from defense to offense.

6.6 SWITCHING STANCE

As mentioned earlier in this book, it is important to train and develop all techniques on both sides of the body, including left and right stances. This will increase the amount of opportunity to land techniques if one is being able to deliver effective techniques from both stances. It can also be difficult for the opponent who may not be used to having techniques from both sides. An example of this can be seen in boxing games, where many orthodox fighters have a hard time against a "south-paw" fighter because they have not experienced these techniques. Switching stances can also be used to distract the opponent just before one attacks. By switching stances just before the attack, the opponent is forced to re-adjust its position, thereby creating an opening for the attack. Switching stance can also be used in defensive "escaping" motions which create distance and angles for counterattack.

6.7 STRENGTH AND FITNESS

Another very important aspect of self-defense and fighting is strength and fitness. While there are many experts and specialists in this field, it is important for an individual to have a working understanding of one's own strength and fitness level and how to develop them to compliment one's technical fighting skills and strategies. For this purpose, it is important to look at the types of physical strength and fitness required for fighting or self-defense. These can be broken down into three categories: *physical strength*, *cardiovascular fitness, and flexibility*. It is important to develop all three of these attributes at all stages of one's development, whether one is a beginner or an expert.

6.7.1 PHYSICAL STRENGTH

A. Weight Training

There are many methods for developing physical strength. The most common are weight training and body weight exercises. Weight training is one of the most popular form of strength training and is used by professional fighters from all types of combat sports. Weight training allows the athlete to effectively isolate muscle groups as well as target and develop different parts of the body. It is important to tailor the weight training to compliment with the activity one is doing (i.e. How much weight? How many repetitions? And at what speed?). For example, lifting heavy weights with slow repetitions can cause muscles to react slowly and fatigue easily which is counterproductive to fighting. It is also important to note that even though most weight training involves isolation of specific muscle groups, it does not always allow for strengthening of all the supporting muscle groups and stabilizers. Thus, only building muscle mass does not necessarily provide effective strength for fighting or self-defense. For these reasons, it is important that weight training as a strengthening exercise must be done under the supervision of a professional weight trainer who can tailor the program to meet the specific needs of fighting and the competition format. Bigger is not always better!

B. Body Weight Exercises

Another method of strength training is using body weight exercises. These exercises utilize the natural weight of the body as a kind of weight training. These exercises include push-ups, sit-ups, leg raises, pull-ups, muscle-ups, and any other body weight exercises with their variations. These kinds of body weight exercises allow an athlete to build physical strength and muscular endurance simultaneously. They also involve the use of all stabilizer muscles and supporting muscle groups, thus creating whole body strength which is directly applicable to fighting or self-defense. Body weight exercises help in developing a strong abdominal core and supporting back muscles. A strong "core" is necessary for any kind of contact fighting as it facilitates stronger punching, kicking, and striking techniques while also making the body more resilient for receiving such techniques.

It is recommended to include several types of body weight exercises in one's training program for any kind of combat competition. It is also important to focus on increasing repetitions and difficulty of exercise as one's strength and endurance improves. For example, push-ups can be done with variations of hand positions such as hands closed together, hands under the shoulders, and hands wide out of the body. Each of these variations will change the muscular focus of the exercise, creating muscle groups with a wider range of dynamic strength, and a stronger muscular support structure. As the strength increases, change to one handed push-ups and vertical push-ups (i.e. hand stands) to further increase the strength. The two-handed push-ups become easier when sufficient strength is achieved and one can do large number of repetitions. Push-ups can also be done on the fingertips to help increase grip strength and wrist strength. As one's hand strength increases, three finger push-ups using both hands can be done with the body weight resting on the thumb, index, and middle fingers of both hands. One's hand strength can further be intensified by doing three finger push-ups using only one hand.

The same strategy can be used with pull-ups starting with regular two-handed pull-ups, with the hands closed, and hands wide out, increasing repetitions as they become easier. One can then increase intensity by moving to one hand pull-ups and eventually to muscle-ups. Muscle-ups is where a pull-up is finished by pressing the body weight above the pull-up bar and straightening out the arms.

Sit-ups and leg raises are also very important exercises and should be a regular part of the training schedule. They focus on strengthening the abdominal muscles which are the "core" of the body and are used in all aspects of fighting or self-defense. These can be intensified by holding some weight on one's chest when doing sit-ups and having someone push one's legs down on each repetition during leg raises.

6.7.2 CARDIOVASCULAR FITNESS

Cardiovascular fitness can be looked at as the body's ability to keep up with the physical demands of fighting. These demands are not only in the form of exerting energy for punching, kicking, striking etc. but also for receiving physical blows as well as mental and emotional stresses that can also tax one's energy output.

Cardiovascular fitness can be built through regular exercises such as running or swimming or other prolonged intensive activities. In order to build the kind of cardio fitness required for fighting, running or swimming program must be tailored to best replicate fight conditions. Jogging alone is not sufficient, sprinting must be included at regular intervals to help replicate the bursts of energy needed in a fighting situation. For example, running 400 meters and sprinting 100 meters and then repeating this as many times as possible. The same can be done with swimming, alternating a regular speed swimming with full speed swimming.

Another important aspect of fighting is the mental and emotional stresses. The stress during any fighting situation usually involves a strong feeling of anxiety which can lead to a burst of adrenalin. This in turn, can cause an extreme feeling of fatigue, loss of energy, and ability to fight effectively. A similar sensation can be experienced when hit with a hard blow or when overwhelmed by an aggressive opponent. In these situations, it is essential to maintain composure, regulate breathing and stay focused during that moment. This is very difficult to do if one has never been in a similar situation before.

It is very important that training for any fighting competition or self-defense situation must include training under stress. Contact sparing rounds against different opponents, timed extended rounds of striking drills with counterstrikes, combinations and any other drills that replicate the stresses of fighting. This kind of training will lessen emotional responses and avoid any bursts of unwanted adrenalin. During this kind of training, it is important to focus on regulating the breath and keeping the mind focused. In other words, techniques, strength, and fitness alone cannot create a strong chance of success in a fighting situation, one must be trained to overcome and manage the physiological responses to the stress and chaos of a real fighting situation.

6.7.3 FLEXIBILITY

Flexibility is an important aspect of training for any fighting competition or situation. It can make executing techniques easier and more effective and can also help in preventing injuries during training. Improving flexibility should be a goal for all fighters and martial artists and should be included in all training sessions. It is suggested that stretching exercises for all the major joints, muscles, tendons and ligaments, starting from the neck and all the way down to the ankles, feet and toes. Stretching must be done before and after all training sessions.

Joints should be rotated in both directions with smooth movement and muscle groups, tendons and ligaments should be stretched with established stretching techniques targeting specific muscle groups and connecting tissues.

It is also highly recommended to adopt yoga or similar practices as a supplemental discipline when training for any contact fighting competition or situation. In fact, it has been proven that practicing yoga can be beneficial in the areas of flexibility, mental focus, and breath control for competitors of all contact combat sports.

6.8 CONCLUSION

The formula for success in any fighting competition or situation is complicated and requires a very solid foundation with layers of hard work and dedication towards perfection and excellence. The truly dedicated fighter, Budoka and warrior must develop powerful and balanced basic techniques, master movement at all distances, blend these techniques into seamless evolving combinations, solid defensive skills, master the minor deviations of timing, and remain calm in the face of aggression and danger.

The overall goal of this book with all its illustrations, explanations, and video demonstrations is to provide a solid foundation and the directions one can apply in any situation, whether in a combat competition, self-defense or any other dangerous, scary or intimidating obstacle or challenging situation. This book and its illustrations are written under the guidance of Shin Gi Tai, Judge and let one decide with the wisdom of its three eyes and build the fortitude to stand unshaken in the face of difficulty and adversity.

TRAIN HARD! AND ALWAYS GO FORWARD IN LIFE. WASHOY MAEDA!! (TOGETHER IN HARMONY, GO FORWARD!!)

www.ingramcontent.com/pod-product-compliance
Lightning Source LLC
Chambersburg PA
CBHW051256110526
44589CB00025B/2848